Water

Fasting

Activating Autophagy and Increasing Mental Clarity

(Unlocking a New Level of Self Confidence and Body Positivity)

Rosalie Reulet

Published By **Ryan Princeton**

Rosalie Reulet

Water Fasting: Activating Autophagy and Increasing Mental Clarity (Unlocking a New Level of Self Confidence and Body Positivity)

ISBN   978-1-998769-38-4

No part of this guidebook shall be reproduced in any form without permission in writing from the publisher except in the case of brief quotations embodied in critical articles or reviews.

Legal & Disclaimer

The information contained in this ebook is not designed to replace or take the place of any form of medicine or professional medical advice. The information in this ebook has been provided for educational & entertainment purposes only.

The information contained in this book has been compiled from sources deemed reliable, and it is accurate to the best of the Author's knowledge; however, the Author cannot guarantee its accuracy and validity and cannot be held liable for any errors or omissions. Changes are periodically made to this book. You must consult your doctor or get professional medical advice before using any of the suggested remedies, techniques, or information in this book.

Table Of Contents

Chapter 1: Get Charge Of Your Life By Fasting With Water Fasting

Fasting isn't new in any way in the realm of imagination. Fasting has been practiced throughout the ages due to necessity, as for instance, in the instance of our hunter and gatherer ancestors or for reasons of religion, such as Islams fasting during Ramadan or Catholics abstaining during Lent.

And it has always been beneficial to improve our health and wellbeing. Nowadays, people are suffering more and are more susceptible to heart disease more than ever. Our ancestors and those only the past few generations didn't have the same issues with obesity that is currently affecting us.

This is fascinating because today there are a lot of advances in medicine and technology which can aid in treating people who are sick. This is the problem when you're taking preventive steps, you'll stop illness and diseases from arising for a significant portion of the time. There's no need to visit the doctor to receive medication. However If you fall sick, now you require medication or antibiotics to get rid of the illness.

The prevention of something occurring (such as sickness and disease in this instance) is more effective than trying to find a cure that can help diminish or eliminate the symptoms of the issue. Think for a second, what's more profitable-- preventing a problem or curing a problem?

If, for instance, I give you a fishing pole you're done. It's a once-off sale and now you're able to keep yourself fed for the remainder of your life by fishing for a fishing trip on your own. Also, I'm able to sell this fish direct. This is the most convenient option for you, as you won't need to spend any additional effort in catching the fish by yourself. It also benefits me since I will continue to sell your catch and make money from it throughout your life.

All of this is to claim that corporations don't take care of your health, they care about your money. If it's more profitable for them to promote a drug that can treat your illness instead of encouraging you to take the situation in your own hands it's likely that it's what they'll be doing. We're here to say that you definitely can be in charge of your health and wellbeing. Is it the most simple thing you've done? It won't, but the payoff is definitely worth it.

What exactly is water Fasting What is it?

I'll go over the meaning of water fasting in a moment however it's important to know the distinction between intermittent and water fasting. Intermittent fasting is gaining popularity in recent years and should not be mistaken for water fasting as there are distinct differences.

Intermittent fasting means that you fast periodically from intervals. For instance, you could do 16 hours of fasting each day, or fast for 24 hours or 1-2 times every week. The practice of fasting in general has been gaining popularity due to the health benefits as well as weight-loss benefits it could bring.

But, a more intense form of intermittent fasting is called water fasting. Water fasting is basically the most intense form of intermittent fasting. When you're doing water fasting it's important to first decide how long you'll need to fast for. If you're a beginner it could be 12 hours or 1 day, but if you're more experienced people have fasted for up to thirty days (2)! While fasting it is not possible to eat foods, and the only thing you consume is water.

The concept behind water fasting is easy to understand in the beginning however it can be very difficult when you're not familiar with it. The benefits are worthwhile, however. The people who do it experience weight loss and mental clarity. they can rid their bodies of toxins by taking a break from food for a certain amount of duration. In terms of positive health effects, lets dig into the details and find out what water fasting could help you...

Benefits of water Fasting

What makes water fasting so effective is the numerous health benefits you get through it. Here are some benefits of water fasting:

Benefit #1: Weight Loss

This is among the major benefits that water-fasting has to offer. Because you won't consume any calories when you're doing a water fast is a fantastic method of losing weight. In addition, it's also a great way to develop self-control so that you're not as tempted by salty and sweet foods in the near future.

It's not unusual to lose anywhere from .5-1 1 pound each day drinking water. There's a lot more to water fasting other than just losing weight, but read chapter 8 for additional details about how you can utilize water fasting for losing weight and maintain it.

Benefit #2: More Self-Contol

Do you find yourself purchasing food items from the supermarket that you realize you shouldn't? Do you remember things like cookies, chips and Ice cream? Do you then discover yourself eating these foods at times when you shouldn't?

If you have trouble with this, as most people drinking water will definitely assist you. We all lack discipline in eating and nutrition. It's tempting to succumb to our desires and cravings to eat.

While you're fasting you'll be exercising the highest level of self-control. Don't think about eating food that isn't healthy You won't be able to eat anything! This is sure to help strengthen your willpower and will enable you to become more adept in delaying the gratification of more rewards in the future , rather than continuously consuming immediate pleasure. When your fast is complete it will be easier to refuse certain food items at the store or stay away from eating unhealthy food attending a gathering with your pals.

Benefit #3: Eliminate cravings

One of the most common symptoms you encounter during your fast is the feeling of craving. It's essentially a last-ditch attempt by your body to go to previous routine. Be tough and refuse to give up!

If you can make it through your urge to indulge in junk food then you'll be free. You'll not be tempted by sweet foods any more. This is an excellent thing because you'll be the sole decision maker of what you take in, rather than let your feelings dictate the shots when they want to.

Think about how difficult you have to fight your urges and resist the temptations! It takes a lot determination and willpower to be certain. When you've shown the cravings that you're boss with your fast to drink water and they'll be thinking twice before attempting to get you back.

Beneficial #4 Improved Cardiovascular Health

Cardiovascular disease is on the rise today. More than 600,000 Americans are eating a healthy diet each year to avoid cardiovascular diseases (3). The reason for this is largely to have to do with the fact that the majority of Americans do not eat a healthy, nutritious diet. The average

American consumes fast food 4 times a each week (4).

The fatty food consumed are clogging our arteries, creating plaque. In the years of sitting and carrying around extra weight, plaque buildup is bound to catch up with our bodies eventually.

This is where fasting with water can be beneficial. It will give your body the opportunity to clear its own pores and begin breaking down the plaque that has been accumulating within your arteries. It will also assist you in getting back to a healthy weight which could help reduce the levels of cholesterol and your blood pressure.

Imagine waking up energetic because your blood flow is flowing in a fluid way, just like it should! It's definitely possible, and all it takes is an determination to boost your health by the practice of water fasting.

Benefit #5: More Energy

Have you ever had large portions of food and feeling sluggish afterwards? The reason is due to the fact that your body needs to transform the carbohydrates you eat into blood sugar, so they can be used to generate energy.

When the blood sugar of the food you ate has been consumed the energy levels decrease. This is typically the time when your body starts to feel hungry and signals that it's time to take another bite of food.

The best part of fasting is the fact that it causes your body becomes more efficient in making use of fat as energy rather than carbs. What's the reason? Fat is digested more slowly than carbohydrates are.

To allow your body to utilize fat as energy source it has to be transformed by your liver prior to it is used to generate energy. This process of breaking it down fat and using it to produce energy is a more secure process than the one used for carbs, which could quickly rise and cause a crash in glucose levels.

That means you'll have an energy stream that is steady through the entire day. Naturally, it will require some time for your body's system to adapt as it's used to getting energy through food instead of storage of body fat.

Benefit #6: Greater Mental Clarity

Another benefit you could experience by fasting is better concentration as well as mental clarity. If you've had difficulty being able to concentrate, or have trouble thinking clearly or have experienced mental fog Fasting could aid you. This mental fog is due to fluctuating blood sugar levels.

If you are a regular eater of lots of starchy carbohydrates in your diet, then you blood sugar levels are likely to go up. As we all know, the food you consume will be lowered, which means the blood sugar levels will eventually plummet. This causes your brain to feel slow and sluggish.

As we've mentioned previously, when you're the water fasting, your body will become more proficient in using fat as fuel. Fat is a far more stable fuel source than carbs and helps keep your mind focused and focused.

Benefit #7: Detoxification

If you're a student, working in addition to school and an extended family You're probably a very busy person. It's hard to pay attention to your health and wellbeing when you're focused on managing other obligations. Your body is also busy as you are.

It is constantly trying to digest food and fight illnesses and infections. When will your body get the opportunity to cleanse itself? It's not unless, obviously you do a fast.

If you are fasting by eating a low-calorie diet, your body gets an opportunity to relax from the constant need to take in and process the food that you consume. This is a great way to let your body concentrate on other tasks including cleansing itself. Your body could show different signs of detox, so make certain to read the next chapter to find out more about it.

Do not worry it's a good thing, as it's a signal of your body cleansing itself of all the toxic substances that have accumulated within your body. In the end, less contaminants in your body is an improved functioning immune system and will allow your body to be more in a position to fight off illness and infections.

You'll also feel more relaxed and feel more energetic. It's essential to maintain your body's cleanliness when the fast is finished by eating a balanced diet. It's not going to do much good to cleanse yourself just to indulge in junk food and then re-intoxicate your body when the water fast has ended.

Chapter 2: The Symptoms Of Fasting Water

One of the most important aspects that will occur when you go on a water-fast is that the body will be cleansing itself. If you've consumed lots of junk food over time, the junk food has stored up in your body and it must eliminate the waste. Fasting with water will give your body the chance to cleanse itself.

Naturally the fact that these toxins are removed from the body will not be an enjoyable experience the first time you attempt an exercise program. Every time you go on an exercise it's different. Some days you'll be energetic even though you've not eaten for 3 days. At other times, you could feel ill on day 3.

Before you start Don't expect every water fast to be a complete disaster when your first experience with it is difficult. Don't also expect every water-based fast to give you unlimited energy. In that regard, there are a few common signs that are experienced by people who are you are fasting for water. In the first place, be sure to consult your doctor or doctor before beginning any kind that of fasting.

Common symptoms

The first symptom is bad breath.

It's one of the most annoying issues to tackle because who doesn't like having bad breath? In comparison to the other issues you may be experiencing, bad breath does not seem to be a problem at all. Here are a few reasons for this:

The reason #1 is Salvia within the mouth

In the course of your daily meals, your body produces more salvia. The salvia can help eliminate one of the bacteria present in your mouth. But, if you're not eating your body will produce less saliva in your mouth.

This means you won't break down the bacteria which causes bad breath. The best method to reduce bad breath during fasting is to ensure that you're eliminating all food particles that have been trapped inside your mouth. Make sure you're brushing the surface of your mouth at least two times each day.

But, this will not be enough to accomplish the task. It is also necessary to begin flossing your teeth even if you're not already doing so. Many foods tend to become stuck places between the teeth areas that our toothbrushes aren't able to reach.

Flossing can help you reach those difficult-to-access places. If you're not a fan of the standard string of floss, you can purchase the floss picks from the local store. They're a lot simpler to use than standard string floss, and makes the habit simpler to master.

The reason #2 is that there are bacteria in the stomach

We do not only suffer from oral bacteria which could cause bad breath, however, we also have bacteria within our stomachs which could create this problem as well. The stomachs of our bodies contain digestive fluids which help digest the food we consume. Naturally when we're on a fast the fluids don't contain any food products to break down which can lead to bad breath.

There's nothing you can do to stop this. The most important thing to avoid is eating food items like onions garlic, garlic, and other foods well-known for giving people bad breath prior to beginning your fast. In addition there's not anything else to do. So be ready to be faced with a little bad breath during the water-fast!

Symptom #2 White Filament on Tongue

As with the smell of bad breath could be among the most unpleasant, but not painful symptoms you be able to manage. It's possible to notice an opaque white layer on your tongue while you're fasting. Do not be concerned There's a rational explanation for the reason for this.

The tongue contains four distinct types of papallies--filiform, circumvallate and the foliate. Filiform isn't equipped with taste buds, as the other three types of papillae. It's a different protein known as Keratin is found on the surface of the papillae.

If you eat food and eat, the food you consume will be absorbed by the keratin layer and disappear when you take a swallow. But, when you're on a fast there is no food. So, the keratin does do not have anything to rub off and remains there. This is what causes you to develop an opaque white layer in your mouth.

You can purchase a tongue scraper or the toothbrush to clean your tongue to reduce this. There's nothing alternative to do for it, and it's mostly an inconvenience that you'll be faced with when you're trying to complete the water fast.

Symptom #3 Headaches

Headaches are another issue you may experience while your body is cleansing itself after a water fast. There are a few reasons the reason for this. The primary reason is that we are drinking less water in general.

If you're running an exercise that involves water the only water source you'll receive is from drinking. In general, however the water you drink not just from the fluids that you drink, but also from the food you consume. We often forget how much water is found in certain food items, like vegetables and fruits.

It's possible that we don't notice it while eating these kinds of foods but you'll likely be aware of it once it's gone. Make sure you're drinking a sufficient amount of water throughout your water fast to ensure adequate nutrition and to compensate for part of the fluid that you're not getting from not eating anything.

Another reason that you could suffer headaches while on a water fast is due to the low levels of blood sugar. If you're not fasting it means you're not consuming glucose, which means your body will need to store energy to generate fuel. It might take some time for your body's system to adapt to the glucose you're feeding it from your diet, and what it's stored.

The brain will receive less energy than normal and can result in headaches. In time, however your body will become better at using its energy stores effectively and will adjust to the fasting routine. In the beginning, it might be difficult to manage however, don't abandon your fasting completely since headaches are a frequent manifestation.

The symptom #4 is rashes Pimples, Bumps, rashes or Other Irritations on the skin

If you're following your drinking water-only fasts, you could be noticing that your skin is worse for a period of time, even though you're supposed to improve your skin's appearance and feel healthier. It is possible that you breakout with pimples or develop an itch. The reason for this is because your body is cleaning itself through the biggest organ that is in your body, the skin.

Don't be concerned when it occurs to you. The itching can be quite uncomfortable It's actually your body's method of flushing out by pushing the toxins into your skin. When the irritations and rashes are gone, you'll have an improved and healthier skin if you follow healthy, nutritious diet after you've finished your water fast.

5th symptom: Aversions

If you consume a lot of sweet or salty food items, you're likely to experience cravings throughout your water fast. A few studies have shown that sugar is as addicting, if not even more so than hardcore substances (5)! Imagine a drug addict who can't take his medication for a week.

There's a good chance that he'll experience withdrawal symptoms that are difficult to deal with. If he's solid and does not break his back, he'll be free of his addiction to drugs. Imagine it as that you remove your body entirely from sweets.

Your body will revolt and fight. It's not able to take it on. It'll urge you to give in and eat something that's full of sugar. Be able to resist this urge and remain stronger than the urge. If you resist the urge, you will be able to find freedom on the other side and the craving is no longer a factor in your life.

Symptom #6: Dissolving in the Bathroom

It could be among the most extreme signs of fasting. Always stay to the side of cautiousness. If you're throwing up violently and you think it's time to stop your fast, and by all means take it. You'll be able to do it to do it again in the future.

Take a moment to think about what it is that causes you to vomit. The reason your body is throwing up is because something is inside your body that is causing harm to it. Your body can rid itself of harmful substance, bacteria, etc. by flushing it out of the body through vomiting.

When you're on a fast the body is cleansing itself of toxins. One one way to accomplish this is to throw up. When you do have a bowel movement, you instantly feel more energized. At other times, you're having to urinate all night long and you wonder whether it will ever cease.

It's important to recognize the difference in this sign. If you're throwing up in a frenzied manner for hours at a time and you're not feeling well, it's probably time to stop the fast. However when you throw up once or twice and feel immediately better and feel better, then you may be able to keep going with the fast. Of course, use your best judgment.

Symptom #7 Shaking

It is possible that you start shaking when you are on the water fast too. This isn't as bad as vomiting or headaches in the bathroom, but it can cause a lot of discomfort to manage. The reason that your body may shake during a fast is because of hypoglycemia. It is simply a matter of low blood sugar.

In the normal course of eating carbs the glucose enters the bloodstream. A hormone known as insulin will be released to aid in the absorption of the glucose into cells, so that the glucose can be utilized to generate energy. The glucose that remains will be stored in your muscles or liver as glycogen.

As you'll be on a fast which means you'd probably not eaten anything for a few days. The body needs energy to function, therefore the pancreas releases the hormone glucagon. It helps in the breakdown of glycogen stored into glucose, which can then be utilized for energy.

In normal circumstances the body is used to receiving a constant supply of glucose from the foods you consume within your daily diet. It's not used to break down glycogen, which is why it might require some time to adjust that could cause shaking. In time your body will adjust and improve its ability to use glycogen stored in the body to power itself, instead of using glucose that you get from your diet.

8. Symptom: Excessive Emotion

The last water fasting symptom that you may experience is intense emotional reactions. Fasting not only helps remove toxins from your system, it may bring your emotions that you've been avoiding out to the surface. Perhaps in the past, you've relied on food as a method to deal with tension or tough moments you had to endure.

Since you've been eating a strict diet, you'll stop hiding in food to hide the emotions. They'll be exposed. This is a great thing. Fasting can help you let it all out and out in the open.

Most important is how you handle those random emotions that you could encounter while fasting while drinking. There's no need to suppress these feelings by not noticing them just let everything out! If you're feeling like crying then go ahead and let it out. If you're looking to kick and scream then shout and kick.

If you can let all these feelings out then you'll be closer to discovering your real self. Once you've let everything out There are some options to help you calm down and get back to your normal state. You can take an extended walk and reflect on your feelings and the way you felt when you let it all out, or soak in a relaxing bath. The most important thing is to realize that it's fine to feel intense emotions while fasting, let them flow and be in the moment rather than trying to enclose them back.

Moving to the Next Level to ensure You'll be successful by setting your Goals

What is water fasting got to have to do with setting goals? Actually, quite a lot according to the research! Think about it this way: how many people realize that they should exercise and eat healthy for a better condition? Everyone knows this!

Then why do very few people are in a position to improve their health? The answer lies in the mindset. Being able to think clearly will enable you to do what you must do in order to succeed in your fasting in water.

It's crucial to set goals that ensure that you keep your eyes and focus precisely where it ought to be. Unfortunately, when you set goals, the majority of people either fail to do it or make a mess of it up. Just 3% of people have their goals written down (6) In the 3% who write them down, which percentage do you think can maximize their efficiency?

However, the majority of people do not ever bother to write down what they want to achieve. They simply keep the idea in their heads as a vague idea. Here's the exact procedure you must follow to ensure that you succeed in achieving your goals every single time:

Step 1: The first step is to record your goals using a pen and paper. This makes the goals you're aiming to reach tangible instead of a thought in your mind.

Step 2: Next you must write down your goals with the present time, as the case of getting them achieved. The subconscious mind is the only one that can recognize the present, so you need to write your goals in a language that your brain is able to comprehend.

Step 3: Establish an exact date to reach your goals. This is a real commitment and creates a sense of an urgency to reach your target. If you don't establish an appointment date, what is the benefit to you? Maybe you'll be able to accomplish it someday when you're ready? Imagine you were getting married , but you didn't decide on a date on when your wedding would take place. What a joke!

Step 4: Write your goals so that you can easily view them. What's the point of having to record your goals and then put them in a drawer somewhere you won't ever see them?

Set your goals in a place where you'll see them constantly in the background of your desktopor an index card inside your wallet. You can place them anywhere you think of to keep them in the forefront in your head.

Step 5: Write down your goals each day and at night. It may seem boring, but it does the trick. Your mind is always searching for solutions to problems. If you write your goals down before sleep, your mind will get to work trying to figure out how to reach the objective. After that, you'll record your goals at the beginning of the day. In this way, you'll keep the determination to achieve your goals throughout the day.

Step 6 Do share your goals with others. It's a little intimidating, but it'll pay off when you've done it. Share the news with your family and friends. Tweet it to social media. Don't be intimidated to go on the market and obtain what you truly desire.

Many people fear that they'll be seen as failures and hypocrites if they say something to that someone, but don't take action to prevent it from happening. It's even more frightening to not do anything and be cautious because you're scared of what other people might consider.

I learned this in high school, when we were voting on the school's favorite. One girl told me that I should cast my vote for her, and I informed her that I would. Then, a second girl told me, "No Thomas, vote for me!" So right then and there, I changed my vote to make everyone happy.

One of my classmates intervened and firmly told me I needed to choose who I wanted to and quit trying at pleasing everyone. He was right. No matter what you do to accomplish in your life there will be people who criticize. Put yourself out there and achieve what you desire!

Step 7: Set several goals. Don't be afraid of setting several goals at each time. You are able to make as many goals you'd like. If you aren't able to accomplish any of them on the date you have set and you don't meet it, pick a new date when you'll be able to achieve the goal.

Step #8: Establish goals that are not health or health goals. Yes it's a book designed to enhance your overall health and wellbeing But, it is important to establish goals for all aspects that you live in. Why not set goals?

Here are some examples of how to note your health-related goals:

* I have completed a 5-day water fast before May 15 in 2018.

* I weighed 130 pounds on June 18, 2018.

* I will lose 10 pounds in body weight by October 30, 2018.

Note how effective the goals are when written in the present past. Imagine you say that I'm going to reach 130 pounds on the 18th of June 2018, 2018. So why not appear as if you've already reached the target?

Naturally, those kinds of goals are known as outcome goals however they're not the only kinds of goals that exist. They also have process goals. These are the tasks you must do to reach the goal you want to achieve. For instance Here are some of the actions you'll have to perform to accomplish your goal of finishing the 5-day water fast

* Determine a date and set a date for when the water fast is scheduled to occur.
* Take at minimum 3 liters of water daily.
• Plan an exciting evening routine that you can follow throughout every day during your water cleanse.

For every one outcome goal you've set for yourself, you'll want to include at minimum three process goals that accompany it. Imagine your outcomes and your process goals as the shape of a mountain. The summit is the desired outcome you'd like to attain, it's the place you'd like to go. The remainder part of it is the procedure, it's what you'll have to accomplish to get to the summit of the mountain.

Should You Concentrate On Your Outcome Or Process-related Goals?

In terms of your goals, should you concentrate more on the objectives for the process or your goals for the outcome? This is a difficult decision to make because there must be a balance between both. If you're focused only on the end result, then you'll forget about the process and will fail to perform the tasks required to complete the task. However If you're only concerned about the outcome you'll doubt the motive of this in beginning.

So, you should focus on the end-goal as soon as it is reasonable while focusing on your process goals only when it is logical. Let's say, for instance, you're feeling demotivated to keep going in your water-fast. It's day 3 of your fast, and you're feeling some of the signs of fasting and all you would like to do is surrender.

In times like these It is crucial to keep in mind the end goal. This will provide you with the drive to keep going by doing the fast even when you're not feeling up to doing it. If you only fast for a short period that's simple, then you'll never reap the benefits that drinking water can bring. When you think about it, the thought about your goals for the process will only bring back all the tasks you must go through and accomplish to reach the conclusion of your water fast.

For instance, if you are thinking to yourself, "Oh shoot I still have 5 days left on this water fast, how am going to get through the most of it?", it's unlikely you'll be able to finish the task. But, if rather say to yourself "No. I'm bored of my sluggish life, and I'm determined to improve my energy and health in order by the end of summer I'm going to do what I'm confident of, even when I'm not feeling it. I'm determined to be healthier than I have been and nothing will hinder me!"

Do you feel the difference? Do you find that recollecting your goals for the end result doesn't inspire you to complete the task? This is due to what is known as the principle of pleasure and pain. It states that people engage in behavior because of one of two reasons: fear of pain, and the potential for enjoyment.

Take a look. Did you ever have an unpopular job for more time than you ought to have? I have done it. I was desperate to find an opportunity to work, any job, for crying to the world, therefore I made an application to numerous establishments. The only one to contact me was a pet shop, so I accepted the offer at $8.60 an hour, and then left on my way.

It was true that I didn't like my job in the least. The reason was not because the pay was low, it was because I was interested in fitness and health more than pets. However, I was at the job for two years before quitting. The reason I didn't quit earlier was because I was scared of what could occur:

* How can I pay for rent?
* Could you be able find a new job?
* Could I afford to pay for food?
* What do my parents think about me not being employed?

This is the reason I decided to continue working at the job I hated. Insufficient funds to cover the basic needs is a bit scary. But, when it comes to fasting in water it is unlikely that there will be any consequences that can be attributed to failing to complete the water-fast. It's unlikely that you'll be removed from your home or not be able to purchase other essential items when you don't do the fast.

So when you're trying to reach the fitness targets you have set, you should concentrate on the possibility of enjoying yourself. Imagine how great it will feel being healthy and filled with energy. Imagine the compliments you'll receive from family and friends. This will motivate you to keep going even where you're not sure you are able to do it.

The Best Way to Find Your Why
Apart from noting down your goals and objectives for the process One other way to inspire yourself is to identify what is your "why." It's an explanation, or several reasonsfor why you'd like to meet your fitness and health goals. It's the fundamentals motivation will get you fired up. For every outcome goal you're working towards, consider what the reason you'd

like to reach the target. Find at least 30 reasons to reach your various outcomes objectives. Examples:

Outcome Goal: I will weigh 150 pounds at the end of June, 2018.
Why?
* I'd like to have the old clothing to be able to accommodate once more.
* I'd like to become healthier.
* I'm trying to demonstrate to myself that I am capable of doing it.
* I'm trying to be a role model in my home for my kids.
* I would like to feel energetic throughout the day.
* I would like to feel confident in myself.
* I'd like to be more attractive.
* I would like to look nice in a dress that is slim fitting.

Once you've thought of every idea you're able to think of Then, you can think about asking "why" for your initial "why's" 3-4 times. This will help you get closer to the thing you really want. The "why's" the you

think of are the most effective and inspiring of all. For instance:
My motivation is simple I'd like to feel more attractive.

Why am I trying to look more attractive?
I'd like to be more noticed by men.
Why should I want men to pay attention to me more?
I would like to be invited to join additional dates.
Why would I like to be invited out on further dates?

So I could be in an intimate relationship.
So, the primary reason to look more attractive is because you're looking to get into an intimate relationship. Keep that in mind and the other motives, even if you're not motivated to accomplish what you have to do.

Personally I like to write all the reasons I have for why down on a piece of paper. Then, I tape the piece of paper on my wall, right over my computer, where I always see it. When I don't feel motivated to do anything, all I have to do is glance at the paper and I'll immediately be reminded of why I must do my best.

Here are a few of the motivations that motivate me to improve my health and fitness:
*I don't wish return to work at the pet shop.
* Being ridiculed because you can't lift 200 pounds bench.
* I do not want to have to accept orders from my boss.
* I would like to be able do what I want when I want, and with whom I need.
* Being criticized because I'm skinny, and being told that I'd "blow out with the breeze."
* I would like to realize my fullest potential.
*I don't wish stress over my finances.
* Not receiving any offers to play in the NCAA basketball tournament.

* I didn't give my all for basketball. I'm not doing similar with my fitness or in my work.

* I was offered a job that pays $8.60 an hour, after I completed my college degree. Writing these things out inspires me and I'm certain that it's exactly the same thing for you! Write down your goals, your motives for doing it, and then get to the task!

Chapter 3: Transitioning Into A Water Fast

Do you need to jump into the water fasting if not done before? Perhaps. If you're the type of person who goes from eating a lot on the one day and then not eating anything the next day, then you can go ahead. But, I'm willing to bet to accomplish this, you'll fail badly and won't be able to complete the water-fast.

The best option is to switch to water fasting. I would suggest spending approximately one month transitioning into fasting in water. This might seem like a lot of period of time, but it's time well-spent. This will allow you ample time to gradually adjust to fasting , rather than trying to make the transition for a few days after that jumping right into a 3-day fast.

It isn't easy going from eating three meals per day, and then not eating at all. There are several various ways to go into a fast for water. The second is to gradually cut down portions in your food. For instance when you're for a whole month in the transition period, you can break it up by following the following pattern when you're eating a typical breakfast, lunch and dinner:

• Week 1. Cut down the amount of breakfast you eat in calories by about 250.

* * Week 2: Cut down the calories of your lunch and breakfast by 250 calories per day.

3. Week Three: Forget about breakfast and cut down on the amount of your dinner and lunch by 250 calories for each meal.

* * Week 4 Forget breakfast and lunch and cut the portion of your meal in calories by about 250.

* * Week 5: Begin your water quickly.

Implementing a transition phase this way will allow your body to adapt to eating less calories. It's a much easier change for your body and therefore you're more likely succeed with it. Each week you'll striving to be at the top of the amount you're fasting, which will oblige your body to adjust.

Another method to consider can be intermittent fasting. Like we said earlier intermittent fasting is just taking a break every now and then from eating. There are numerous methods of intermittent fasting available in our day-to-day life However, we'll be simple and not eat breakfast, and work towards a higher level from there.

Here's how to set up our four-week transition into intermittent fasting with water in the case of eating a normal breakfast lunch, dinner, and breakfast:

• Week 1. Forget about breakfast and eat your usual lunch and dinner.

* * Week 2: skip breakfast and cut down on the size of your usual lunch by half.

3. Week: No the breakfast or lunch.

• Week 4 Avoid lunch and breakfast, and cut the amount of your usual dinner by one-third.

Week 5: Begin your water rapid.

This method of transition is a little more forceful than cutting down on your portions. The first step is cutting out breakfast. This isn't easy for some to deal with. If this happens as the scenario with you, you can try to get through it or use the other approach. If you've never skipped breakfast prior to it may take a few weeks in order for the body become familiar with it.

You can also mix both strategies to help you transition into the habit of water fasting. Here's how you can go about it if you're eating regular breakfast, lunch and dinner:

• Week 1, Forget breakfast and cut the portion that you eat for lunch by about 250 calories.

2. Week 3: Avoid lunch and breakfast.

• Week 3. Forget lunch and breakfast and reduce the portion of your meal in calories by about 250.

* * Week 4 Begin your water rapid.

This combination approach can allow you to start your water fast one week faster than any one method alone. But, you shouldn't feel pressured to do things in a hurry. It can be exciting to start by doing a water-fast, and you're likely looking forward to seeing how it goes and the benefits it could bring you. I strongly suggest to take your time, breathe deeply, and slow down.

It's not good to jump into water fast only to end it earlier than you planned to. You can be able to regroup and attempt to do it again but it's mentally draining. You could end up until you can't consider the value of going back to the drawing board. You must keep going. It isn't easy to fast in water however, anything worth doing isn't easy to attain. Recall your reasons from the previous chapter, and keep moving forward even when it begins getting tough (because it will become tough at certain points).

What Foods to Eat During Your Transition Time

If you're using one of the two methods of transition there is no need to make any major changes in regard to your diet during the initial three weeks. In the final week you'll be able eating more liquid-based foods to prepare your body for an extended period of fasting.

In the beginning you'll probably only eat an enticing meal So changing what you eat shouldn't impact the overall calories. Here's a list of healthy foods to aid you in transitioning to a water-only diet (not an exhaustive list):

* Mashed potatoes
* Soup
* Vegetable broth
* Fruit
* Vegetables
* Smoothies

Of of course, there are other options to eat similar to these, however the basic idea is to consume liquid or soft food items that can be easy to digest by your body. If a week of just eating this type of food is too much for you to handle and you're not sure what to eat, then you could eat more solid food for the first one or two days during the last week in order to make it easier. I would suggest however that you at least for the last three days before you begin your fast you only consume liquid-based food to make the beginning of the water fast less stressful.

What should you drink during The Transition Period?

If you're drinking lots of other beverages in addition to water The transition phase is an excellent moment to let go of these drinks. In the final week of your transition phase all you'll need to consume is drinking water. You may drink occasionally refreshing water with sparkling or herb teas when they are low in calories.

In the initial three weeks of your transition period, you'll need to gradually eliminate all beverages that aren't water. For example If you're using soda as a source, you might want to begin abstaining from soda drinking every day until you've eliminated the beverage. In the following week, you could concentrate on reducing the amount of drinks you're drinking, such as orange juice.

Many people are mistakenly convinced that juice is healthy for their health, however, the majority of juices are loaded with sugar. Even if you prepare your own juice using fresh fruit, you'll have to remove it from your diet as it will be permitted during the fast.

The most important thing to remember is to devote approximately a week gradually removing every beverage you're drinking.

If the only drink you're taking other than water at the moment is soda, you may need to take several weeks gradually to get rid of it , rather than only one week. Here's an illustration of how to accomplish this in the event that you're drinking 16oz of soda every day:

1. Day One: pour 4 ounces soda and dilute the soda using 4 inches of water.

* Day 2: Same as day 1

Day 3: pour 8 ounces soda and dilute the soda using 8 ounces of water.

* Day 4: Same as day 3

5. Pour 12 ounces soda and dilute the soda by adding 12 8 ounces of water

* Day 6: Same as day 5

• Day 7 Drink water only

Of course, if wish to make life more simple to manage, you could extend the phase of transition and extend it. If you're taking in more than 16-20oz per day, then you may be required to extend the period by a week or two due to necessity.

How do I Water Fast

Once you've completed your stage of transition, you're in the right position to begin your actual fast. What you'll do during your water fast is easy to do--you just drink water and absolutely nothing else for the majority part.

Although the concept is simple, the execution of it over a long duration of time might not be. This is why you should ensure that you adhere to this specific step-by-step guideline to maximize your chances of success:

Step 1: Decide the length of your water speed. Will Last.

Before you begin an intense water fast, the primary step is to determine the amount of time you'd like to stay on the fast for. If it is your first time undertaking an intense water-based fast, begin with something as simple as 2 or 3 days. It is possible to take a half day in case you had trouble during the transition phase.

The most important thing is to not be hard on yourself. You can always try more than one water fast later, and build on the work you've already done. Most of the time, people are looking for instant results.

It's possible that they will jump straight into a 15-day frenzied and be a failure. It's okay to gradually build toward 15 days (or extended) fast. Do not feel pressured to leap right into a long-term time frame if you don't think you're likely to be capable of completing it.

Begin with just a few days. Learn a bit to your name and gradually increase the duration. After you have completed a one-day water fast, then move to an overnight water fast. After that , move on to three days and then on and so on. Whatever you decide to do be sure to know the length you would like the fast to last prior to the date.

If you've reached the conclusion of your time-span and you believe you can easily continue and continue, then absolutely, take it up. Create a new duration of time you'd like to continue for, and set that as your new goal. However when you're experiencing severe symptoms and wish to stop the fast , take action.

Your body knows you better than anyone else. simply because you've decided to do three days of water fasting doesn't mean you need to stick with it until the final. Be aware. Keep in mind this: just because you didn't succeed this time doesn't mean you'll be able to do it again at some point in the near future. Get yourself back up and ready for the next time.

Step 2: Be aware of Your Schedule

This is perhaps the most crucial aspect of water fasting. It's not possible to be able to anticipate the entirety of what's going to take place while you're drinking fast but you'll need to have control over all of your timetable as you can. The purpose of a water-based fast is to have an unwinding state both physically and mentally, so you're able to let your body cleanse its internal organs.

If you are working in a challenging job that is physically and mentally what will your body perform in cleaning itself? It's not going to be. So, you must get rid of your schedule and go home to relax. If you've got some left over vacation time, take advantage of it to have the chance to enjoy a "stay-cation" and finish your water quick.

If you are employed in a position where you are unable to get several days off in a row, you can start by starting small and finish your water fast on the weekend. The idea of getting away from the crowd and relaxing at home can appear to be a minor thing but it's actually vital. Consider it.

Do you think your colleagues are aware whether you're running the water fast? Not a chance. They'll be eating right before you during lunch breaks. Being surrounded by customers eating is likely encourage you to end your fast. This is a bad idea.

Even if you have in a cubicle is still mentally draining. You do not want to waste your time and energy on your job when you could have saved it. This means you may need to wait a longer before you can complete your water quick, or you may be required to plan things for a bit longer however it's worth the extra effort.

Step #3: Remove Potential Distractions

The next thing to think about the potential distractions that may encourage you to eat when you're in your home. An excellent example is T.V. When you are watching T.V. an advertisement for fast food might be on and things might be going well up until the point where things be completely destroyed by a snarky commercial.

It is possible that you don't consider a simple commercial. It's possible to believe that commercials aren't affecting your life, but studies show that they definitely have an impact (7). Naturally, if you're not hungry, watching ads for food probably aren't much of a problem. If you've not consumed anything for several days, all of suddenly, that commercial could be extremely appealing.

The best option for yourself is to sit down and watch prerecorded TV if you're able to do so or to not be watching T.V. for the duration of your speedy. This isn't worth it. Instead , what you can do is stream something similar to Netflix and Hulu.

Again, if you choose to stream Hulu be extremely watchful because there are ads on Hulu. Even if you're on Netflix it is important to be aware. If you're watching a program with lots of food or even those eating food, you'll be enticed to eat something you should not. It's obvious that watching cooking shows is not a good idea. A documentary-type show (nonfood connected) is a great idea.

Another thing to take into consideration are your loved ones. It is possible that you eat meals with your family members or with others who are most likely not going to be on an exercise with you. In this situation, you'll have to be able to isolate yourself from your roommates and family when they are eating. There's no intention to be socially isolated here, but it's too risky to giving into the scent of food.

These are the kind of things which you'll have to plan in advance to ensure you have the greatest chances of achieving success. If even a tiny fraction of you worries that feeding your cat could result in a fall and burn and burn, then find someone who will feed your cat while you're watering quickly!

Step 4: Make a Plan of Your Plans for Your Fast Water Fast

If you're planning on in your home for the majority of your fast, you'll require something to keep your mind busy. If you're not engaged or distracted, do you know what you're likely to be thinking about? That's right, food! It's also the last thing you'll need to think about while conducting a water-fast and it's best to anticipate the activities you'll be performing all day.

The best way to begin is to consider some of your favourite activities or activities or. They should be enjoyable and non-strenuous things, but is there something you've done previously that you've totally lost in? It's about hours and hours that passed by without you even realize it was happening.

You didn't take a meal, or perhaps you did not go to the bathroom because you were so involved in this task? This might be an entirely different experience for individuals. Whatever the activity an excellent idea to perform during your water quickly.

Here are some suggestions for how you can stay staying at home on your water fast

* Video games (of course, play ones that don't make you feel stressed!)
* Read books
* Check out a new series on Netflix
* Draw or paint
* Light exercise, such as walking outdoors or stretching
* Meditate
* Listen to podcasts
• Listen to the music

These are just a few ideas to help you get your mind going however, you'll need to at a minimum have an idea of the activities you'll be engaging in throughout each day in order to stay occupied.

Step #5: Create a Something You're Looking Forward to Later in the day.

Another method to keep your mind free of thoughts about food, is to create something thrilling to look forward to later on in the day. Develop an evening routine you'll be able to follow each day throughout your water fast. Here's a good evening routine that you can follow:

1. Stretch and stretch for 30 minutes
2. Take a walk outside For 30 minutes
3. A warm bath while listening podcasts or music for 30 minutes
4. Book reading: 30 minutes

Of course, you are able to choose to do what you want but I suggest you have an action plan that will last for at least one time of an hour or two hours. This may seem like a lot, but just think about when you were a child at Christmas or any other holiday you were excited about. What was your mood the night prior? The excitement was such you were unable to get to sleep! The thought of what you would consume was probably the last thing you thought of!

Step #6: Complete the Water Quickly

You've put in plenty in planning and preparation to this point and the additional time is well-worth it! You've prepared your body for the highest possibility of being successful. Now all you need to do is stop eating.

It's not eating whatsoever here. There are no supplements, limes or lemons, and gum, no juice or milk, etc. The only thing you can drink is water.

It may sound boring and dull, and this is exactly the case! The concept to drink soda and eating sweet pastries is way more appealing than drinking plain Jane water! Keep in mind that drinking water is the primary goal for the whole fast! This is the way to get your body into the ketosis state and reap the incredible benefits that water fasting can bring. Keep going, since the reward is well worth it!

Chapter 4: What To Do Swim Out Of A Water Fast

What you do after your drinking fast can be the single most critical aspect of the whole water fasting procedure. The longer your fast lasted the more crucial the process of letting go of your fast. At the end of your water fast , your stomach will be sensitive and soft.

If you finish your fast with many foods which are hard to process, it could cause digestive problems like stomach upset or perhaps vomiting. Of course , thinking about what foods to eat in order to finish a fast or how long you'll need to take to get out of a water-based fast is probably not the first thing you're thinking about but it should not be. What to do to end an intense water-based fast should be the main focus!

How Long Do You Have to Wait to get out of a water Fast

The length of time you'll need to devote to transitioning out of a the water fast is largely due to the length of time the water fast you did. If you've been through intermittent fasting and have fasted just 12-24 hours, as an instance, there's not any requirement to break your fast. You are able to come out of your fast and eat whatever you want however it's recommended that you eat healthy.

But, when it comes to fasting with water it is likely that you will be fasting for a period of time that are a little longer than 12-24 hours based on the level of experience you have. This will allow your body more time to cleanse itself , and your stomach will shrink somewhat as well.

Additionally the stomach will be more sensitive to foods that you consume when you break your fast. Here's a helpful timetable that you can follow to figure out the length of your transition is:

Length of the Water Fast Transition Period
3-4 days, 1-2 days
5-6 days - 2 days
14 days, 1 week
The basic idea is to consider how long your speed, and divide the length in half. This will determine how long the transition out

of the water fast needs to be. To clarify it, this is how much duration you'll have to spend following your water fast has been finished. As an example, suppose you were planning to do an entire water fast over one week. You shouldn't be able to in a fasting state for 3.5 days before beginning your exit from the fast during the rest time. It would take you a whole week drinking water, and then take the next three to four days transitioning out of the water fast.

What Not to Eat when you are transitioning out of a water Fast

What exactly is it that you should not eat after you've completed the water fast and beginning to transition back to regular eating habits? Right off the bat there are a few things to stay clear of are dairy and meats.

Many animal products are highly processed and it is possible that you will be able to consume the foods you like without any issues however, remember that you haven't eaten in many days. You are in an extremely delicate state right now, and all those chemicals and processed ingredients could make your body uncomfortable due to the fact that it has spent the last couple of days cleaning its internal organs.

It's not just limited to animals, but you must be wary of processed food items when you break an edgy water fast. Of course, it's best to be avoiding processed foods in any way you can and it's particularly crucial when you break the fast. This is the reason that you should avoid animal products, as they can make your stomach feel uncomfortable after it has had cleansed itself of the toxins.

Imagine the feeling you get after having your teeth cleaned by the dentist. Your teeth are spotless fresh, and sparkling. You probably don't want take a bite after having a meal since it can ruin that sparkling shiny feeling that you feel! It's similar to how your body feels. It's spent the last couple of days, or even weeks sanitizing itself and isn't going to let you cause harm to your body by eating junk!

Another thing to stay clear of is fats. Although not all fats are harmful to your health. Certain foods like avocados and nuts are actually quite healthy. In this situation, however it is best to stay clear of eating any kind of fat.

The reason is that fats are difficult for the body to digest and need more effort your body to break down the nutrients and then process them. This is called the thermogenic effect of food and it's a fascinating concept to consider if you're seeking losing weight. This is due to the fact that your body burns calories in order to process food you consume!

But, if you're coming from a fasting period it's something that you'll need to be wary of. It's not a good idea for your body to expend more energy than it needs to use to digest and process the food you're eating. This is why you'll want to stay away from eating protein and fat in the course of completing your water quickly.

You might be surprised to learn that you'll have to stay clear of foods high in protein as well However, protein is the highest thermogenic effect of all macronutrients (protein carbs, protein as well as fat). This means that your body is required to work harder to digest proteins rich foods and you'll want to make things easy to your system.

What Foods to Eat When You're Out of Water Fast

Once you've figured out what foods you shouldn't eat during a water-fast What exactly can you eat in order to break the fast? One of the most beneficial things that you can eat to get from a fast is food that has lots of water.

One great example is juice smoothies. The liquid makes it easier to your body's digestive system as well as the fruits and veggies that make up the smoothie will have structured water. Water that is structured the body to replenish itself with water. This is distinct than bulk water which needs to be transformed in your body into structured water to be utilized.

Here's an alkaline list of fruits and vegetables that you can use to make smoothies and juices:

Fruits:

* Watermelon
* Mangos
* Pears
* Passion fruit
* Cantaloupe
* Grapes

Vegetables:

* Kale
* Collards
* Spinach
* Chard
* Cucumbers
* Celery

Take at least half of an hour to a whole day drinking only drinks like juices of fruits and vegetables and smoothies. Then, you are able to begin to consume soups made that contain bone or vegetable broth for a few days. Then, you can transition to eating fresh fruits and veggies throughout the transition time.

That's everything there's to. You should be eating vegetables and fruits when breaking a fast with water due to the fact that they're full of water and are easy to digest. It's possible that you'll be hungry and want to devour all the food you can find after the fast has ended However, be mindful of your eating habits. Your stomach will be grateful numerous times over for taking it easy!

Water Fasting to Lose Weight

One of the primary reasons to be interested with water-fasting the fact that it will help you lose weight. It's true that if you do not take in anything, and only drinking water then you'll lose weight.

However, you will not be able to live all the time without eating any food. So it's essential to know the body's functions with regard to burning fat in order to be capable of completing the water fast and remain weight-free for the long haul.

Why do we need energy?

Your body performs a range of various tasks. It is required to absorb food, breathe and circulate blood, among others. Each of these tasks requires energy. The question is where our body obtains the needed energy needed to keep itself in good condition?

It's all in the food you consume! Foods contain calories, and calories are merely an indicator of energy. If you consume something with 200 calories, but I consume something with 300 calories, then I'm eating more calories than you do.

However, you must make use of this energy. If we do not, our bodies keep the energy that is left (i.e. it will store any leftover calories) in fats for later use. It can be a bit depressing to consider.

Why aren't our bodies able to remove all the calories we consume? Why is it that they have to be in the form of fat? In fact, if the extra calories were not stored as fat, then you and I may not be around this moment...

How Our Ancestors ate and. What we eat within the Modern World

Then when food was scarce, it was a luxury. Our ancestors didn't have the luxury of going to a fast food establishment and order a hamburger or fries. They also couldn't get milkshakes,

milkshakes, or even. They had to look for their food, or track for it.

Like us, they didn't know the place where their next meal was going to be coming from. So, when they did discover foodsources, such as a huge buffalo, for instance it was feast. All the extra calories that our ancestors were likely to consume in the days ahead would be stored in energy to be used as they hunted for their next dinner.

This was good for our ancestral ancestors. They didn't have as much fat since they didn't have as many chances to overeat like we do. If they did indulge and eat, it was a great choice because the stored fat could be useful when they couldn't to get food for a long time.

In today's world the world is very different. It is possible to eat a lot every day, even at any meal we want. We don't need to look at animals that we can hunt or something similar.

If we are hungry, we could take a break and eat a meal. Here's the issue arises. When you were younger when you had to be restricted from eating because there wasn't a fridge that you could walk into and prepare sandwiches.

There's nothing that forces us to fast or make us accountable. If we'd like to eat more food, we easily have the ability to. There's not much in our modern times that could stop an individual who is hungry from eating. This is yet another benefit of fasting in water.

You'll increase your determination to keep going regardless of whether you have to live like our forefathers did. Things like obesity and cardiovascular disease were not as prevalent at the time as they are today, and water fasting will help you return to eating more in the same way the way our ancestors did.

Where did my sweet tooth Where Did My Sweet Tooth

As was mentioned previously one of the advantages from water-based fasting is it will assist you in getting rid of your cravings. If you find yourself regularly wanting ice cream or cake for instance drinking water can to get rid of those cravings. Where did they come originally from??

It is possible to think that the reason that humans enjoy salty and sweet foods is that corporations are constantly advertising junk food all over the place and that's why you want to eat unhealthy foods. In reality, you naturally crave these foods, and the advertisers try to capitalize on this natural craving.

The innate desire for sweet and salty food items may seem like a curse however, in the absence of it then we would not exist now. In the past the food supply was limited. Our ancestors had to eat whatever they could find.

A bush with a few fruit on it was okay it would supply calories however not much. But, food items that contain sugar (such such as honey) or salty and fatty will provide us with a lot more calories than we normally eat. This was good because it let us quickly take in more calories and then store the extra calories to use later.

When we ate sweet and salty food, it released feel-good hormones into our brains, such as serotonin and dopamine (8) that signal our brains that we should to consume these foods whenever we could. In the past, when the availability of salty and sugary foods was extremely difficult to find and this natural urge to consume sugar and salt was a positive thing. It kept us alive.

Now fast-forward to today and the overconsumption of salty and sugary food items can do much more harm and damage than benefit to the majority of people. You may recall earlier that studies have found sugar to be as addictive as substances!

This is definitely something to look out for. Everyone needs to be more conscious of when they're planning to consume unhealthy food due to this reason alone but unfortunately, a lot of people are eating like they have no time for tomorrow.

How does your body gain or lose weight?

As I've mentioned before the body requires energy to sustain and maintain your existence. The energy you get comes from food you consume. What determines the amount we can consume before we begin to store foods as fat?

It's also known as your resting metabolic rate , or the rmr acronym for short. In essence, your rmr is the amount of calories you'll eliminate in a single day. In other words when you're burning 2500 calories per day and this is the case, it implies that your metabolic rate is 2500 calories.

A caloric surplus occurs the case when you consume more calories than the resting metabolic rate. The same is true for the example above. when your metabolic rate at rest is 2,000 calories, then when you consume over 2,000 calories,, you'll be experiencing a caloric surplus. A caloric surplus can be described what it sounds like: a surplus of energy or calories.

These are calories that your body doesn't have the need to utilize, and so will keep the excess as fat to be used later. What it means is that if you consume much more than what you burn them off and you start becoming overweight. On the other end of the coin is the caloric deficit.

A caloric deficit happens when you consume less calories than your metabolic rate. For instance that your rate of metabolism is 2,000 calories but you consume under 2,000 calories per day, you'll be experiencing a deficit in calories. This implies that your body requires more energy than what you're providing it with, and will have to source the extra energy source from somewhere.

The body usually draws on the fat stores in order to obtain the energy it requires for its continued functioning. In rare cases it is possible that your body uses your muscles to generate energy. This is only the case when you're in a energy deficit over a long period of time, and you're not doing any exercise or eating sufficient protein.

It's not as common as the publications that promote protein powder tell you to believe! But you might still be concerned as there will be no food even during a long. True but keep in mind the fact that when you are fasting,, your body naturally releases an increase in human growth hormone (9).

This additional human growth hormone can protect your muscles from being used to generate energy when you're not fasting. As you're doing weights (when you're not fasting in water, of course) every 2-3 days and eating sufficient protein (.8-1 grams per pound bodyweight) You don't have anything to be concerned about.

The rumours that you should consume proteins every two hours, or else you'll lose muscle is just that, a rumor. The only thing you should be aware of is that when you consume less calories than what you're burning then you're in an energy deficit and you'll start losing weight. This is an excellent thing since being in a caloric shortage is only the way for your body can shed weight!

Here's an easy outline of everything:

Samantha has a metabolic rate of 1,600 calories.

* If Samantha consumes 1,600 calories per daily, that's the recommended level, and will neither gain or lose weight.

* If Samantha consumes over 1,600 calories in a day, Samantha will have a state of caloric excess and will begin increasing her weight.

* If Samantha consumes less than 1,600 calories per day, she'll be in a deficit of calories and will begin losing weight.

How to Find Your Resting Metabolic Rate

How do you determine the resting metabolic rate is? There's a formula that is very easy you can employ to find out the exact formula-

Bodyweight in pounds x 13= resting metabolic rate

Let's suppose for instance the following: Samantha weighs 123lbs. Here's how she can determine her metabolic rate at rest:

123 x13=1,600

Then it's easy! Now Samantha realizes that in order to shed some weight, she'll need take in at least 1,600 calories. But how many less calories should she consume?

Determine the speed at which you Are Looking to lose weight

Okay Now Samantha is aware that she has to consume under 1,600 calories to shed some weight. What number of calories should she take in? Sure, she could eat a little less than 1,600 calories, or suppose 1,500 calories, but that would only be a fraction of what it takes to move the needle in the near future.

On the other hand you could also adopt a drastic approach when she's not fasting in water and cut down her daily calories up to 800. Remember that 800 calories a day is how many calories she eats when not on a fasting day. This number of calories could make her lose weight fast, but it's not sustainable over the long run.

It's the reason I recommend finding the right balance between not having to cut calories too drastically however, you can have cut them back enough that you can make noticeable change to begin losing weight.

Since there are about 3500 calories in a pounds of fat (10) Aiming to have a cumulative deficit of 3500 calories per week is logical. If you multiply 3,500 times 7, you'll have 500. This means that you'll have to maintain an average daily loss of calories by 500 to shed a pound each week.

Utilizing Samantha to illustrate time:

Resting metabolic rate = 1,600

1,600-500=1,100

This implies that Samantha must eat 1100 calories a day to lose about 1 one pound every week.

Yes, but how do I apply this to water Fasting?

Naturally, when you're doing a water fast, you're not taking in any calories. That means that you'll create an enormous caloric deficit which can lead to huge weight loss. It is possible to lose as much as .5-1 pounds or more each day while water fasting. The reason it's vital to determine the resting metabolic rate of your body is that it will determine how much you'll need to consume even when you're water fasting.

If someone begins an exercise program, they'll be experiencing a deficit in calories and will begin losing weight with no difficulty. The problem comes up when the person is able to come off of the water-based fast. What does it mean to you to do if you water fast only to return to the normal routine and eating unhealthy food?

It does you no good! You'll end up gaining all the weight you lost through the water fast. If you're aware of your rmr, you'll be aware of how many calories you'll must consume to keep losing weight after your fast is done.

The advantage of the water-fasting method is because you'll be creating a significant caloric deficit throughout your fasting period, you'll likely to eat levels that are maintenance or even an surplus for a couple of days and yet lose some weight. It is all dependent on the amount of weight you'd like to lose each week and how often would like to perform water fasts.

Do not do more water-fasts within the timeframe your body is able to handle and don't get too obsessed that you attempt to shed all of excess weight in just one week. It's not like you gained all the weight in a single day, so do not try to shed it all in one go.

One example is to determine that you'd like to lose 3 pounds during the weeks that you water fast and gain 1 pound per week during the times when you don't drink fast.
The amount of time you fast for will affect the amount of food you'll have to eat the remainder of the week to meet your goals. If, for instance, you take part in a drinking program and shed 2 pounds it means that you have remaining five days to shed an additional 1 pound needed to meet your weekly goal.

3500 calories per kilogram of fat / 5 days = 700 calories

That means that you'd be required to consume an energy deficit of around 700 calories daily during the remaining five weeks to shed that extra kilogram.

The Most Important Takeaway From Water Fasting to Lose Weight

Do diets generally work for the majority of people who attempt them? They don't! The reason for this is that people are looking for an immediate fix. They want to transform in a matter of minutes.

It is the reason why they adopt irrational actions in order to reach their objectives. They'll make decisions that don't work in the long term and will put themselves in pain for the length of time they can endure it. When they're unable to take it any longer, they stop their diet, eat in a frenzied manner and gain all of their weight back.

After they feel better at themselves, they attempt an alternative diet plan, and the cycle begins all over. This is called the yo-yo diet, in which you lose weight only to increase it, after that, you lose it and gain it back, etc. To stop this cycle of viciousness individuals must not view dieting as something unpleasant that you're eager to finish. Instead, it is important to adopt changes to their lifestyles.

The simple act of changing your words to say, "I'm on a diet" or "I'm making lifestyle adjustments" will have a significant effect on your psychological well-being. Take a moment to think about the word "diet. What thoughts come to thoughts?
When I think of diet, I am thinking of changes in the short-term. I imagine someone who is on diet, and that means they'll eventually have to go off their diet. Think about the word changes in lifestyle. What does this mean for you?

According to me, lifestyle change refers to a complete and complete shift and a completely new way to do things. This is the way to take on the water fast and weight loss. You can't, of course, follow a water-only diet for the remainder of your life therefore, you must include it in the lifestyle changes you are making.

Perhaps that lifestyle change involves taking a water fast at least every quarter or every month and then you do it for a lengthy time to be. Then , the rest of the time you're not doing a water fast eating nutritious and healthy food items that nourish your body and provide your body with energy that it requires.

Do you mean you'll eat healthfully all the time? Of course there's no guarantee! Imagine if your life changed to eat healthfully and clean food 90 90% of all the all the time. This is a lot more achievable and viable! It's still possible to enjoy delicious food during family events and celebrations.

What you do not wish to do is to begin drinking water and then immediately return to eating the same way you did before. After you have gained the weight back, begin another water fast , and then jump back to snacking on junk foods. It's similar to the yo-yo diet method I discussed in the past, but the long-term outcome will not be very good.

Be aware that simply losing weight isn't the end goal. It's not a good idea to shed weight only to gain it back. It is important to lose weight, but know it won't come back. The only way to accomplish that is to include drinking water and eating healthily as a change in lifestyle which you will continue to do for the long haul.

Chapter 5: Tips And Tips To Make Fasting Water Easy

Absolutely, fasting on water can be extremely challenging, particularly if you're familiar with the idea. The thought of going for on a whole week without eating isn't easy to comprehend. The first thing to be aware of is how amazing our brain and body are at adapting to the environment present.

To demonstrate this an academic at Innsbruck University of Innsbruck conducted an experiment on his assistant in which the professor made him wear a pair of glasses that reversed his eyes (11)! The entire world was turned upside-down! The assistant initially was unable to walk and struggled with regular tasks like getting into a seat, grasping an object, or walking up the stairs.

But, around one week, something fascinating began to occur, and he began to adjust! In reality, within 10 days was normal to him. His brain was adjusting to the new surroundings.

Imagine being the subject of this study. It's going to be a bit difficult initially, wouldn't you think? You may even ask you, "How will I ever be able to get over this?" But eventually you'll adjust to the circumstances and make it through it.

This is also true for fasting in water. There will be difficult times that you'll need to endure however, if you keep going you'll adjust to it and the reward will be waiting when you come back. Whatever you decide to do, don't quit!

Try again until you get the you are comfortable with it! If you must stop a water speed faster than you'd like keep in mind that you could come back later and try again however, do not give up for ever! It's the only chance of losing. That being said there are a few things are you able to do to ease your fasting more manageable:

TIP #1: Get Started Small Intermittent Fasting

The idea of fasting for 3 days or for more than a week can be extremely difficult. Don't be compelled to jump straight into a three-day water fast if it doesn't make you feel at ease doing it. If you'd like to splash your feet into the pool and experience the experience is like in a water fast beginning with intermittent fasting.

When you are on an intermittent fast it is simply taking breaks from eating. There are a variety of methods of intermittent fasting that are available and if you are interested in learning the more details about these methods, make sure to read my other book about intermittent fasting.

At this point I'll break down a couple of well-known techniques. The first involves fasting each all day, for 16 hours, and then eating the remainder during the week. Here's how you can organize your food schedule:

* Noon Meal #1
• 4:00 p.m. 2nd meal
* 8:15 p.m. 3rd Meal

In essence, when you have finished your meal around 8:00 it is the time to begin your fast. Then you'd end your fast on the following day around noon. You can alter the times at which you're eating however you'd like. If you adhere to the principle of fasting for 16 hours a day each day and you'll be ready to go.

The alternative is to fast for 24 hours a couple of times every week. You are able to start your fast at any time you want and when you begin the fast, you aren't allowed to take food or drink for the following 24 hours. As an example, suppose you finished your last meal on Wednesday around noon.

This means that you won't be able to have the next food item until Wednesday noon. The main thing you need to do with this type of fast is sleeping during the most difficult portion of your fast. For instance, if discover the 8 hour mark of the 24-hour fast to be the most difficult, you can time it so that you're getting ready to go to bed about the 8 hour mark of your fast.

Try intermittent fasting for a month to check how you adapt to it. It's a great way to prepare yourself for water fasting in case you're not quite ready to go all-in.

Tip #2: Eat the organic Apple Cider Vinegar Prior to Bed

A couple of tablespoons of apple cider vinegar can provide a significant benefit to you when you're fasting. But don't be concerned, it won't force you from your fast , nor will it take off the burning fat states called ketosis. The acid in apple cider vinegar can be described as carboxylic meaning it has the ability to enhance the absorption by your body of minerals.

One of the biggest issues many people face when they are fasting for water is mineral absorption. It is possible to lose a significant amount of minerals during fasting, and even more minerals are flushed away when you drink plenty of water, as you ought to be. Consuming apple cider vinegar can assist in maintaining the mineral balance.

It can also assist to maintain your blood sugar levels. If the blood sugar level is going between high and low and up, you're more likely to feel a craving. The more frequent cravings you have and the more likely you'll be to indulge in a binge and crash. Naturally, this is something you'll want avoided as much as you can. Organic apple cider vinegar can assist you in doing just that.

Tip #3: Himalayan Pink Salt

The next day, take 8 ounces of warm water and one teaspoon Himalayan pink salt mixed into the water. The primary reason you should have your water be warm instead of cold is because lukewarm water can aid in detoxifying your body more efficiently. It will also not cause as severe of an "shock" on your body when you first wake up in the morning.

It is Himalayan pink salt can help to provide you with a complete list of minerals aren't consumed by your diet due to fact that you'll fast. It could help reduce blood pressure and assist to maintain your electrolytes in a healthy balance.

Tip #4: Take a cold shower.

It can be a challenge however, try it and see how you feel! If you're unable to take a full bath cold, after you've finished the warm bath, make it off and then stand in it for as long as you're able.

A cold shower can lower the levels of cortisol in your body . It will also aid in waking you up. And not only that, your hair and skin will feel fantastic! A refreshing shower can aid in preparing you for the next day So take a shower.

Tip #5: Go to an Chiropractor

In the course of cleansing your body, plenty of toxins are getting rid of your body. This could interfere with the normal functioning in your nerve system. A visit to a chiropractor while you are on the water fast is a great way maintain your nerve system functioning correctly throughout your fast.

It will allow the proper flow of neurological energy to the tissues and will put your body into the best position to to recover itself. This isn't necessary however it could assist if you're struggling finish the quick.

Frequently Answered Questions

How much water should I consume every day?

There's no set amount of water that you should be drinking throughout your water quick. The most effective thing you can learn is to pay attention to what your body is telling you. It will tell you that you're thirsty. it's a signal that you're in need of more fluids.

It's not an advanced science at all but it's an effective method to determine whether you're drinking enough fluids. Another method you can use to check if your water intake is how your urine looks. If your urine appears yellow, it's an indication that you're dehydrated and that you should consume more fluids.

However If your urine is clearer, it's an indication that you're drinking enough water. If you're looking for to know a specific amount you're aiming at, women should consume at minimum 2.5 Liters of water every day, while males are required to drink at minimum 3 liters of fluids per day.

What type of water do I need to drink?

You should drink the most pure water that you could. This means that you'll need to stay clear of drinking tap water since it's full of chemicals and contaminants that eliminate microorganisms, bacteria, and other microorganisms.

It is possible to drink the spring, distillate water or even filtered water if you own a filtering system. These are the most effective options to ensure you're getting the most potent water you can get.

What do I need to take my water from?

Drink your water in glass. Plastic bottles can contain harmful chemicals, such as polycarbonate, phthalate or BPA's. Consuming water in glass bottles will ensure the absence of any chemicals are in a position to be absorbed into your drinking water.

Keep in mind that your body is cleaning itself throughout this fast, and it is important to ensure you're not putting toxic chemicals into your body that could hinder the process of cleansing.

Do I need to drink warm rather than cold?

The best thing to do is drink plenty of water in the first couple of hours you're awake. This will assist to cleanse your body, and also boost the liver and stomach. Following that, it's your decision. Drink extra cold water should prefer, or continue drinking lukewarm or warm water. The temperatures of the water shouldn't be the primary issue, but making sure that you drink the speed of drinking your water is.

How often should you water Fast?

Answers to the question is likely to differ from person to person. The longer your time is the greater your break should last until the next fast. When you're done with your day there's not a limitation on how many fasts you're allowed to perform. Choose a number within an amount of time that you are comfortable with.

Chapter 6: What Is Fasting With Water?

Water Fasting is widely used to help in spiritual renewal and also as a method that many utilize to lose weight. During the water fast people abstain from all types of food, and only depend on drinking pure water or water that has been supplemented with a variety of minerals, vitamins and other supplements, such as branch chain amino acids as well as electrolytes such as sodium magnesium and potassium. Fasting is often imposed for various reasons, including religious, medical or religious motives. One example of fasting with water for medical reasons is that you are required to be fasting for a particular amount of time prior to when a procedure begins. Fasting is needed to shrink the size of the stomach as well as to keep the stomach clear of acid issues when undergoing surgery. Different religions have various types of fasting. Fasting with water is an important ritual in various religions that could be tied to a particular occasion or when a specific prayers to be answered. The duration of fasting varies depending on the specific requirements and religious customs.

The process of fasting with water is very demanding. One must be prepared prior to the beginning of the fast. Anyone who has experienced water fasting will have less trouble in preparing and maintaining the duration in the fast. For those who are brand new to fasting with water the days of the fast are the most challenging, because your body isn't accustomed to being without food. The health and the age of a person is also a factor to be considered prior to beginning a water fast. People with particular health issues should avoid fasting in water, according to their doctor's instructions. Fasting in water has many advantages, however many people finish their fast prematurely because they were not preparing their bodies correctly before the fast started. The length of time you are planning to fast, as well as other factors are involved with preparing your body for an effective fast. It is important to seek assistance from experts who are experienced when it comes to fasting or from your doctor before beginning the water fast because of the health risks associated with not enough preparation for your body prior to the beginning of the fast.

Where did Water Fasting Come From?

Fasting for water has been a common practice since ancient times. A lot of people would fast for religious reasons. Even though people back then didn't have a huge amount of information regarding the dangers of fasting, they often observed fasting to gain spiritual or religious benefits. When our ancestors often fasted They did not need to be as prepared for a fast like we do now, as their bodies weren't subject to the same environmental causes that which our body's are in the present. Their bodies were in good health which made it simpler to prepare for an upcoming fast. They believed in a religion and were extremely sincere about their fasting. They would fast on specific days of the year or month according to their religious beliefs. They also fasted with prayers, in order for prayers to be answered and for healing to take place. According to studies, water fasting is practiced since the beginning of time when humans began walking the earth, yet nobody knows the exact date the time when it was the initial time when the water fast began. Research has shown that humans have evolved to fast whether intentionally or unintentionally, whichever situation could cause.

In the beginning, people looked at fasting in water as a method of recuperating by bringing total rest for the body by cleansing. The people of the time engaged in water fasting and employed it to treat the body when needed. Once people understood the advantages of the benefits of health that it brought, they continued fasting to heal themselves. In the past, people didn't have accessibility to health specialists or doctors as we have now. They relied on homemade remedies to treat illness and other ailments they encountered. Therefore, fasting with water was very popular for a lot of people.

Benefits of water Fasting
The practice of water fasting has numerous benefits to your health If it is done properly. The benefits of fasting with water have been proved over time and many utilize it as a way to manage various body issues. It has been utilized as a universal remedy to cleanse our bodies of harmful toxins, and to free the body of various health problems. No matter if they suffer from medical issues or not, people are able to practice water fasting to improve their the spiritual and physical benefits to their lives and bodies. Anyone who embarks to a water fast the first time may encounter some difficulties. However, once they have mastered fasting in water and is fully aware about how to perform it and how to do it, he is able to enjoy the experience and is able to appreciate the advantages.

If you browse the web today, you will find a myriad of content and articles written by those who fast as well as other medical professionals to provide the benefits of drinking water. With the assistance of expert health experts it is possible to make fasting an ideal practice for those who want to benefit from the wide range of advantages. Given the number of health benefits it is possible to combat various illnesses and to create a healthy balance in the body with fasting with water. The quantity of water you drink will make a difference.

Depression

Dehydration of the body can lead to depression as well as other conditions that are triggered by depression. A lot of people consume water when there is no other drink to take or when they are thirsty. They have a habit of drinking other drinks such as coffee, soda tea, etc. A lot of people are in the habit of washing down meals with soda or a drink that is high in calories. If one doesn't drink enough fluids and dehydrates, it can happen within the body. If dehydration is present, other problems may arise like depression, that is very prevalent. Depression does not just happen because of dehydration. I'm not trying to identify anything by this assertion. I'm just noting that if someone is dehydrated, the risk of being depressed is greater and they should increase their intake of fluids to see whether their depression symptoms diminish. Fasting is a great method to keep the signs of depression at low. Mental and physical ailments have been proven to be cured by drinking water. Once the body has cleared its body of harmful toxins, and has time to rest, it allows the body and mind time to get back in balance.

Depression is caused by many different causes, however water fasting is still effective in treating several of these causes too. In the majority of people, depression may be caused by foods allergies or processed foods as well as eating routines. If you drink water only all the various areas of the body get cleansed, removing the body of any toxic substances. When the physical well-being is improved, one is mentally healthier too. When one fasts, one gets enough time to relax and relax. The mind is free of negative thoughts. It is therefore recommended to start a water-fast after consulting with your doctor of the family.

Detoxification

Detoxification refers to the process of eliminating toxins within the body. If a person is on a water-fast it is a time when the body's detoxification process is exactly the same as the sleeping cycle. The energy utilized during the fast is used to eliminate the body of any toxins that are accumulating within the body. This lets the body naturally treat any area within the body, which require healing. Through fasting with water, toxic substances in the colon, the liver kidneys, skin and lymph glands as well as the lungs are completely eliminated. The body is restored to balance and is in good shape for cell regeneration after all toxins have been eliminated. This helps to maintain a healthy body, and anyone who is undergoing a water fast will have glowing skin.

During the fast, toxic substances are removed in the human body. The body fights cancerous tumors, viruses, and any other waste materials that are that are present in blood. If one adheres to a regular water fast and regularly, they are able to benefit from the many advantages of detoxification. Regeneration of tissues damaged by detoxification within the human body. The process of detoxification is carried out through the skin and lung. It is crucial to do appropriate breathing exercises that aid in exhalation from the lung. When your body is free from toxins anti-aversion result is created towards unhealthy food items and behaviors like drinking alcohol or smoking cigarettes. Additionally, following the water fast it is not possible to feel cravings for unhealthy sugary snack foods and fast foods. In order to lose weight, it's beneficial to perform the water fast to cleanse every month at least to remove toxins from your body and ease any cravings for unhealthy food. You will notice a number of health improvements as your body is cleansed of toxic substances.

Cancer

Cancer is among the most terrifying diseases that affects many people. Studies have been established that fasting with water assists in treating cancer patients. According to research that water fasting reduces the spread and growth of tumors. It helps to stop cancer from growing in the body. Patients who have undergone chemotherapy with a fasting regime that includes water have had relatively few adverse negative effects. Fasting in water can aid cancer patients to quickly recover, since fasting clears the body of cancerous cells. Fasting with water has been proven to be very efficient in removing the body of various types of cancer. The most effective way to fight against cancerous cells is to perform regular water fasts in order to cleanse the body of toxins prior to cancer even begins to develop within the body.

Fasting during water can help in preventing cancer, and can also help in reducing the growth of cancer. Many people do daily water fasts on an ongoing routine to avoid cancer becoming a reality. Based on research and research it has been tested and confirmed.

Arthritis

Arthritis is a condition that causes inflammation that affects joints. According to numerous research, fasting in water can have significant effects in treating osteoarthritis and Rheumatoid arthritis. When you go on an intermittent water fast, it rids our bodies of toxic substances, which can trigger inflammation within the body. This is the reason for arthritis pain. Many people experience relief after performing water fasts, the requirement for medications is diminished or completely eliminated. The intake of water helps to improve the muscular and skeletal systems of the human body. Also, any suffering from pain will be able to ease the pain following the water fast.

Nowadays, people are looking for more information on natural cures due the risks and side effects that are associated with various treatments and procedures. To treat arthritis, it is vital to detoxify that can be achieved by the practice of water fasting. With the permission from your doctor you can easily combat arthritis and other bodily ailments by regularly fasting with water. It is essential to drink sufficient amounts of water to ensure the well-being of the muscles and skeletal system of the body.

Hypertension

Hypertension can be treated by water fasting. According to studies the medically-supervised water fasts have proved to be effective in treating many patients who are in a water fast for a specific amount of duration. This can help lower blood pressure and allows patients to attain the best health condition. While there are many ways to fast, based on specific diets to treat hypertension drinking water is an essential method. Patients with hypertension are able to participate in a water fast , and once they reach an appropriate levels of blood pressure keep it at a healthy level by eating the vegan diet along with moderate exercising. Anyone who is interested in learning more about the benefits of water fasting to lower blood pressure must consult your physician prior to embarking on the water fast. It is essential to inquire with your doctor for the number of days they recommend that you participate in a fast with water and remember that a minimum amount of exercise and complete rest is essential for people who suffer from hypertension.

It is important to talk to a doctor before going on a fast, as certain conditions could have other consequences on the body during your fast. Since you're hoping for your blood pressure to go lower, it's suggested to take as much rest as you can during the fast. Most people experience the best results by following the right way, and with adequate preparation prior to when the fasting begins. If you look through various websites and health websites you will learn about the significance of water fasting to reduce hypertension.

Memory Enhancer

Water is essential for the proper performance of the body in all its aspects. If the body is hydrated with water, it is much easier to regulate every function that the body has to offer. According to research the brain performs more efficiently when it has a limited calories consumed. On a fasting water the body's organs are all better as a result of the process of detoxification. Stress levels are reduced, which helps the brain think more clearly. If one is not stressed, he will be able to keep more information in his memory , and access the information at a speedier rate. The mind gets more clear during a water fast. When you eat a diet that is unhealthy, there is no impact on the health to your body.

If you are looking to improve your memory, it is essential that they learn about the advantages of fasting with water and eating a balanced diet. If you can read the signals your body is giving you, you'll know when you should fast and how you can keep going with your fast to achieve the greatest results. It will also be simpler to sustain the duration of the fast. With the right preparation you will be able to easily handle longer-term fasts and experience more focused than you did before. The changes you experience will increase during the fast in the water, and by being less stressed, you'll gain better health, which helps the brain and improves memory.

Rejuvenation
You'll feel refreshed when you're healthy physically and mentally. Your outlook on life will improve. Fasting with water rejuvenates your spirit, mind and body. It is believed to be among the most effective tools for rejuvenation. You are physically, mentally and spiritually rejuvenated. Rejuvenation concentrates on removing negative routines and adopting new ones to ensure that you always feel refreshed.

Fasting with water aids in the rejuvenation process by removing toxic substances and waste out of the body. When the body is cleaned completely, one starts to react differently to situations in life and also. When a person is free of food for a while and is able to experience physical, mental as well as spiritual recovery, they begin to feel more grateful for the life they have been given. The more time one spends on fasting in their daily routine and experience, the better the outcomes are likely to be.

The tissues that have been damaged are repaired and illnesses can be cured through fasting with water as well. Fasting with water cleanses the liver, colon lymph glands, and various other areas of the body that result in a rejuvenated body. Additionally, blood sugar levels and blood pressure remain balanced following the conclusion during the period of fast. Brain cells are activated after the blood is cleared as well as all waste products are removed out of the body. When the body is functioning, one can be sure to be healthy in all instances.

Premature Aging
Water fasting can have significant effects on premature wrinkles. Age-related signs and wrinkles visible on your face may be totally diminished through the practice of water fasting. Drinkers who consume more water overall can slow the aging process in their facial skin. When your skin is hydrated, it is youthful and plump. Fasting is a way to rejuvenate your body and mind through elimination of toxins and adequate supply with water. The skin is regenerated. The health of your skin can be significantly improved by water fasting. If you maintain your body's hydration the body performs better and the cells within the body are able to get oxygen, and blood flow is kept. When glucose and blood pressure levels are in good shape and a person is youthful.

For many people, emotional and spiritual changes occur when they fast. These changes manifest themselves in the face of individuals who are regularly fasting in their life perspective is altered completely. While water fasting can be effective, it comes with some rules that certain people need to be aware of prior to starting a fast. If someone is severely underweight fasting is not advised. Women who are expecting should refrain from fasting for a long time. Fasting is not advised for diabetics or mothers who are nursing. People suffering from Anemia shouldn't even consider fasting, particularly drinking water since blood cells are extremely limited and their bodies need to make more blood cells by following a proper diet. Kidneys that aren't functioning properly must get approval from their physician prior to beginning an exercise program.

It is possible to conduct a search on the internet, and read more in depth about advantages of fasting in water. With water fasting, you can keep their health in top shape, and also to gain knowledge about the benefits of water fasting, one can participate in online forums or blog discussions. Each water fast is different from the next. It is a good idea to keep a diary to keep track of the way your body reacts to the fasts as it detoxifies and note down the benefits you reap.

Internal and Spiritual Benefits

When someone participates during a water-fast, they are consuming nothing other than water. This lets the body concentrate on burning excess stored fats as well as storing toxic substances. Although it can take time to eliminate of toxins in the body and eliminate them, fasting ensures that the toxins get eliminated faster, allowing people feeling refreshed. When fasting, one's wellbeing is guaranteed through the peace of mind that can be achieved due to less stress levels.

Chapter 7: Fasting Using Prayer And Meditation:

If a person seeks out God or an enlightened power, they're capable of focusing on their thoughts, utilizing their thoughts and thoughts to attain greater concentration and more clear thoughts also. Meditation and prayer can help make your life more enjoyable peaceful, tranquil and can result in higher satisfaction levels. Fasting with water is usually used to get spiritually closer to God or the power of God by sacrificing to abstain from the consumption of drinks and food in addition to water. By controlling their appetites and remaining focussed, they will receive divine guidance when they pray and completing their prayers by fasting.

Fasting For Weight Loss

If the calories we consume aren't being utilized in the day or due to an active lifestyle our bodies convert and store excess calories as fat the body. When we avoid eating solid foods and not changing your lifestyle, or increasing the number of activities that are involved, weight loss can occur since the body has no choice other than turning to fat stores to use as fuel. Thus, when one adheres to a liquid food plan, the body will absorb the nutritional value faster without going through the whole breakdown solid foods. This could allow them to lose weight faster.

Other types of fasting

No matter what the motivations the person is following a fasting program is because of a desire to attain a higher fitness level, to treat any ailments that might be present in their body, to eliminate excess fat efficiently, to rid the body of the impurities, or to serve a religious purpose, where they can avoid eating and concentrate on the sanctity of their religion It is essential for the individual to determine the best method through that they can attain their desired physical and mental outcomes. While water fasting is thought to be among the most effective methods for cleansing the our bodies of toxins, however However, it is crucial for those who are considering it to understand that it's not the only method by which they will be able to achieve the goals they've established for themselves. You can also use other diet plans and fasts to make sure that they can cleanse the body of undesirable excess fat, toxins and bad lifestyles too. On the next few pages of this book , you will find other kinds of fasting, apart from drinking water.

Absolute Dry Fasting

Absolute dry fasting refers to the point at which one begins a period of fasting by eating a diet that is free of food and any liquid, which includes water. Many people refrain from all contact ever with water, such as showering or washing their hands during fasting. This type of fast can lead to faster detoxification and better mental clarity. It takes less time to attain the benefits of a water-free diet. In order to meet the energy needs of our bodies, we is able to reap the benefits faster by avoiding drinking water and food as it allows their bodies to utilize the glucose supply and move swiftly towards using stored fat as the body's primary source of energy. Because our bodies have stored lots of calories as fat, these stores could be broken down and used as sugars to maintain the energy levels needed.

Intermittent Fasting:
If people are inclined to eat healthy, it is thought to be the period when they are not fasting. At simultaneously, if they don't eat even when they are offered and are considered to be in a state of fasting. Although most fasting regimens will ensure that their users are required to avoid eating for a longer duration, there are some options like in the case of intermittent fasting, where individuals would be able to alternate their periods of fasting and not-fasting to ensure they will achieve the required benefits. Because their bodies aren't fully prepared due to medical reasons but they will benefit from

fasting to increase endurance and cleansing their systems and organs, they can follow strategies that allow them to get the most effective results, without harming their system by any means.

Juice Fasting:

Juice fasting makes sure that people are able to reduce the amount of calories their bodies consume, and also helps one be healthier and slimmer and improve the endurance levels. By fasting with juice, one can achieve optimal health and gain the nutrients needed by drinking juices from fruits and vegetables. Juice fasting is efficient and is believed to be more attainable for those who are new to fasting. Juice fasting has the same advantages as water fasting and dry fasting, however, the amount of time needed to reap the benefits is extended. A lot of people prefer to start by an initial juice fast, then move to a water fast since this helps the body prepare for an upcoming water fast. Utilizing fresh fruits and veggies to juice fast our body with antioxidants to combat free radicals within the body, and keeps the body in a state of balance. With prolonged water fasting alone can lead to loss of essential enzymes, and ultimately deficiencies too. When searching online there is numerous recipes to add to the juice-fast.

You can also participate in drinking"a "Smoothie" in which the fruits are blended together and includes the fiber in the fruit, as well as the juice. And even while this isn't considered to be a fast but it helps your body to keep a certain health balance. It is possible to cut certain vegetables and fruits, and then add them into the blender, blending it into the desired consistency and then drink it as milkshakes. For those who are considering a juice fast there are a variety of recipes and books accessible at book stores and on the internet that one can explore to ensure that they don't get bored of drinking the same foods daily.

But, prior to attempting any kind of fasting practice it is essential to know the basics of one's body, and seek the advice from their physician and follow the advice according to their advice. The good thing is that juice fasting methods are recognized as techniques to detoxify the body and are widely accepted as religious practices as well. However, one note of caution is that those suffering with diabetes should steer clear of fasting with juice due to its significant impact on glucose levels in the blood. Also, those with extremely active lives are not advised to observe specific fasts until they are able to unwind and take part in less energy-intensive activities. After that, they will need to make plans for the body to relax and reap all the advantages of the diet.

How Do You Prepare For A Speedy

It is advised to consult your doctor of family to determine if you are cleared before beginning any kind of fast in particular if you suffer from lower blood pressure or have advanced cancer. This is especially important in the event of long-term total or water-only fast. As mentioned in other parts in this guide, it's not recommended that you drink a lot of medications while fasting since the body's chemical chemistry changes and may cause negative reactions that wouldn't have happened.

In the process of preparing for a fast it is recommended to considered the duration you're going to be fasting, and the reasons for your fast. The typical fast will last anywhere from 1 to 40 days. The reasons behind the fast could range from spiritual healing mental clarity, or weight loss. If you keep this thought in your mind,, you can plan your fast better to ensure you have enough relaxation time, which allows your body to take a break. It is easier to complete an intense fast when you are close to your home, and are not surrounded by distracting factors. If your body exhibits indications of needing to rest, you must be able to lay down and take a rest and not work more.

Numerous experts will advise that it is recommended to begin preparations for a fast with water at least 2 or 3 weeks in advance by drinking fresh juice of fruits. This can prepare your body in a variety of ways prior to the start of a fast in water. Juicing prior to the fast, that your body gets habitual to avoiding the consumption of solid foods. Juicing exclusively with fruit juices will also provide the body with the necessary nutrients and vitamins that will aid in maintaining health over the duration of the fast. When you begin the juice fast, the detoxification process begins which can help you be free of other harmful behaviors like sugar, alcohol, caffeine smoking and alcohol.

There are those who think it's not essential to plan the fast by juicing and to eat in a clean way for a few days before they jump into a warm bath fast and cold turkey. This method has been proven to be more difficult, however those with plenty of determination have battled the detox symptoms and persevered. The cold turkey method is more difficult however, sometimes people are stretched for time and are not able to devote a lot of time or cash preparing for the fast.

Signs of a Detox

The process of change is something that all and everything throughout the world experiences but people still tend to be averse to changes. It is important to understand that this is true in the body too. When there are toxic substances in the body, there's also the possibility of change, although it's an adverse change. To ensure that their body is cleansed of these substances, it has to undergo the process of detoxification. While detoxing, there could be various symptoms that can be affected in various ways, some of which are described below:

1. Headaches:

Headaches may be caused by constipation or dehydration, withdrawal and detoxification can be one of the causes for headaches. So, people who experience headaches after fasting should know that the toxins in their bodies have begun to go through the elimination process and they should not be worried. However, if the headaches do not go away following the first 3 or four days of fasting, it is advisable to consult your doctor to confirm that there is there is no other reason for concern. To get the most effective treatment for this detox symptom , just lay back as much as you can and concentrate on prayer and meditation.

2. Flu-like symptoms:

Because the body is experiencing changes, the immunity could be low, thereby exposing to various symptoms that are often associated with flu and cold since elimination of toxins by the body. There are numerous benefits one can reap in ensuring that the contaminants are eliminated in their system. When one knows the signs of detox you can concentrate on the process of fasting while making the benefits of fasting the ultimate objective.

3. Fatigue:

Because the body is feeling the shock of not eating foods that are solid when it is fasting and it is absorbing the stored toxins, the body can slow down and experience the need to relax as it repairs itself. When doing a fast, one might experience signs of fatigue in which they're not able to concentrate on different strenuous tasks, because the body requires more energy in the process of flushing out of toxins. They can be able to cope without more solid food or intake of calories.

4. Diarrhea:

There are many ways which toxins are eliminated from the body, including via sweat, urine, and through stool movements. Since elimination is quick and quickly, the body could decide to flush out toxins as both solids and liquids simultaneously which can cause diarrhea. It is crucial for people to eliminate toxic toxins from their body, it is important to soak replenish the juice or water when diarrhea continues to persist for a prolonged duration of time, to ensure that electrolytes do not deplete and dehydration doesn't occur.

5. Muscular Aches:
Similar to headaches, some suffer from muscle pain during the process of detoxification because glycogen is withdrawn from muscles during fasting. this can cause muscle discomforts and aches. The more severe your symptoms of detoxification are when you fast, the more it is necessary to remove the body of toxins. In a hot bath making use of a steam bath or sauna may help alleviate these kinds of ailments because they help to flush out toxins via sweating, and also heat muscles to ease the pains. Be aware and cautious when you exit the bath and take

your time, since the heat can cause you to faint when you make rapid movement. It is not advised to take any kind of medicine while fasting, as it interferes with the process of cleansing. Your body is trying get rid of toxins and medicines are a major contributor to produce toxin.

6. Sleeping Problems:

Since the body isn't familiar with a life without solid food or solid nutrients, sleeping patterns are difficult, particularly since hormones are out of balance. But, many people who are fasting try to fall asleep when their bodies are calling for it. In times of fatigue, you can attempt to relax or rest, and those who experience bursts of energy, it is possible to perform things with more power. As I've experienced it, when fasting I've had the ability to sleep very well while at other times, I was in a position to sleep for between 4 and 5 hours each night , and have enough vitality throughout the day in order to keep up my workload without issue. What helped me sleep better was to be able to relax using prayer, visualization and listening to audiobooks or nature sounds each night before going to go to sleep.

7. Flatulence:
Although the stomach and intestines remain empty without the foods that they are consumed produce concentrated hydrochloric acid. Thus, they can trigger heartburn, feelings of chest irritation and acidity, and experiencing greater levels of flatulence, regardless of an increase in gas. It should go away within the first few days following the fast.

8. Cravings:
Since food items that are solid are eliminated during fasting, it's more likely that your body will be tempted to indulge in junk food. This is often thought to be the most difficult problem to conquer. Since the toxins are being removed, it becomes difficult to resist giving to the urges. This is when determination, meditation, and prayer are essential. Make

sure you visualize the advantages your body will receive when the fasting process has completed. This will assist you in continuing through the fast.

9. Weakness:

Because of the lack of caloric intake the body could be, and most likely will feel weak during the fast. Since the body is getting water and not consuming calories, it could be due to due to not getting enough fluids. If one is feeling weak, they must drink more fluids by drinking glasses of water because it could be the reason to feel weak. While fasting, it's recommended not to drink an excessive amount of water at the same time, since it can flush away electrolytes that are vital and damaging to the body. If you experience a feeling of weakness, it can lead to feel faint. Therefore, it is advised that if the feeling of weakness is present, to lay down and allow your body to relax. Additionally, it is recommended to review the tasks they're performing to make sure they are able to store all the energy needed.

10. Body Odor And Bad Breath:
During a water-fast the fat cells are released into the bloodstream, and later, they will be eliminated from the body via sweat glands. The body's odor could get worse because the body is cleansing itself. The tongue can also be covered in a white layer that can be removed through the help using a tongue scraper. The breath can also be known to smell offensive in the state of ketosis when the body is able to burn fat as fuel , instead of glucose. It is beneficial to bathe several times per day, floss your teeth more frequently and perhaps make use of crystals as a deodorant. They are available in a majority of health food stores.

The Best Method To Crack A Fast Water Break
As the body has not digested or consumed any food that is solid for a specific amount

in time, it's essential to be aware that the sudden consumption of diverse foods will be difficult to digest by the body and could cause a nutritional shock that could lead to a number of medical issues. So, just like the lengthy preparation one must undertake prior to the beginning of the fast also, it is crucial to plan out their departure in a way that is also well-planned.

So, prior to introducing food items into our bodies, it's essential for the person drinking enough fluids to build up muscles, and also replenish the skin and fibers so that they do not experience the stress of nutrition that may happen without ending the fast. It is suggested breaking the fast by drinking the juice that has been freshly squeezed during in the beginning of the day. On the second day following breaking the fast, one must be able to reintroduce probiotics called good bacteria, and you can achieve this by adding yogurt to one's diet and continue to consume fruits and juices of fruit. The third day, leafy vegetables can be introduced. On the fourth day, lentils as well as beans are recommended to be brought back as protein sources after which other food items can be eaten again.

It is possible to consult an expert in the field of health for example, an dietician, to plan nutritious meals that will keep you well-balanced and healthy after the end of any kind of fast. The new diet should include lower calorie, low fat and high-fiber foods to ensure that the body is getting rid of toxins from your body. It is essential to have an appropriate plan which would have to be implemented by eating foods that the individual likes so that they adhere to it and attain the greatest results when they begin to introduce numerous types of extremely nutritious food items back to their diet. Thus, it is sensible for the person to begin by eating different fruit and yogurt so that the digestive system will begin to function normal as soon as it is possible.

There are a few extremely important safety precautions individuals must pay particular focus on when breaking the fast. Pay attention to your body's signals Take note of your body of crucial factors that one would need to consider when breaking the fast. First, they must be aware of the body's signals to ensure they don't consume too much or not enough food which are vital for replenishing nutrients that the body has lost by abstaining from eating in the course of the fast. It is now easy to stop eating when they feel somewhat satisfied. When listening to your body and stopping when the body is satisfied it is possible to avoid stomach discomfort, bloating, stomach flatulence and weight gain caused by overeating. So, by following this suggestion, it can help your body to recuperate in a healthy way and not damage the digestive system following the break in the fast.

Take your time and chew well. No one would ever think that this is the most important aspect of breaking the fast.

However, as the body is only drinking liquids during the fast and is only processing liquids, it is essential that the person realize how important it is to be aware of the magnitude of stress that the stomach and intestines will be experiencing. It's just normal sense to must chew their food thoroughly and is recommended by medical professionals that one should chew their food properly. Chewing is the first step in the success of digestion. For proper digestion to occur it is crucial for people to chew thoroughly the food prior to swallowing it that will not only help break down food, it also allows the food to blend well with saliva as it is ground between teeth. The saliva of humans is a ptyalin-based acid that can be able to break down particles as they enter the stomach. This can eventually allow an effective absorption rate of nutrition to greater levels that is crucial for fasting to be successful and achieve weight reduction achievement.

Chapter 8: Food And Human Body

Knowing the science behind water fasting is essential in executing it correctly. You shouldn't do fasting without knowing methods and even the reason's. Therefore, let's begin by introducing a little background.

Histories of Fasting

The first proponents of fasting originated from Greece especially Pythagoras who extolled its numerous benefits. St. Catherine of Siena was a faster in the 14th century, and Doctor Paracelsus described it as"the "physician within" during the Renaissance era.

Fasting in various varieties is a renowned tradition that has been carried on across centuries and has devotees who claim physical and spiritual rejuvenation of mind, body and the spirit.

In the past it was a requirement prior to when soldiers went off to fight. Also, it was a maturation ritual performed whenever the male or female was able to reach the age of majority. In other societies, fasting was practiced to calm angry gods and to prevent catastrophes such as famine or flood.

In the majority of major religions of the world the practice of fasting plays an important aspect of their practice and is often linked to forms of self-control and penitence.

In Judaism it is commonplace to observe an annual fast known as Yom Kippur, which is the Day of Atonement. In Islam this holy month known as Ramadan is the time when a fast from sunrise until sunset takes place.

The tradition of Roman Catholicism, as well as in the Eastern Orthodox, a 40-day fast is observed in Lent similar to how Christ did at the end of the desert forty days. There is a reason why women appear to be the primary advocates of fasting for religious reasons, since it was believed to be an act of chastity and holiness.

It was the English Mystic, anchoress of the English and referred to by the name of

Julian of Norwich who lived during 15th and 14th centuries, remained fast for long periods of time because she considered it way to connect with Christ. In other religions the belief was that Gods communicated their divine revelations and visions to the temple priests.

Fasting can also be utilized to express protest against the political system. The most well-known example is the Suffragettes movement, as well as Mahatma Gandhi who was a faster for 17 sessions in opposition to British rule and to support the cause of Indian independence. Although a healthy fast is beneficial, there are those who have gone overboard with the idea of fasting. For instance, consider the instance of Dr. Linda Burfield Hazzard who caused the deaths of more than 40 patients, who she advised to follow an intense fast. The medical doctor in Minnesota was ultimately found guilty of manslaughter, in 1912. She was found guilty in the year 1938. was dead from her strict regimen of fasting.

There were also Victorian women who were fasting and whose claims included that they could live without food. There was also the doctor from the Art of Natural Hygiene Movement Doctor. Herbert Shelton who has claimed to have helped more than forty thousand people in their health issues.

Over the pond in the UK the practice of fasting was seen as a part of the 'Nature Cure' movement which highlighted the importance of sun and fresh air, exercising and positive thinking' to rid onesself of health issues. Fasting was very popular in the 1920s, and in the initial Nature Cure clinic opened up in Edinburgh. Since then, additional clinics focused on therapeutic fasting began to pop up like the famous Tyringham Hall located in Buckinghamshire and Champneys situated in Hertfordshire. Although initially it was regarded as a naturopathic clinic but it has now become recognized as a popular spa in the present day.

Fasting has been proven to treat numerous ailments like heart diseases obesity, overweight, high blood pressure as well as allergies and digestive problems as and headaches. The fasting regimens were tailored to the person's particular needs. It may be a period of fasting that lasts just only a few days or could last for 3 to 2 months. These clinics consider the patient's entire medical history to determine whether they could undergo a fasting program or not. And if they could, the patients would be closely watched.

As time went on and medical technology continued to evolve and getting better the natural treatment for illnesses was discarded with those of the British and was quickly replaced with better medications and more sophisticated medical techniques.

In Germany In contrast, in Germany the popularity of fasting was growing especially due to the pioneering work by Otto Buchinger. Otto Buchinger. German hospitals also conduct fasting weeks as an additional treatment that helps fight various diseases like obesity and blood pressure.

In other regions of Europe like Hungary, Czech Republic, and Austria spas and centers are extremely popular, and offer fasting vacations. The practice of fasting in Germany is known by the term "naturheilkunde," which means the practice of natural health. It's still very popular in Germany because it has been incorporated into medical practices of the present and, therefore, the fasting can be prescribed by physicians to their patients.

In the US the US, fasting is increasing in popularity with millions attempt at fasts like Intermittent Fasting and Water Fasting to keep their weight and health. This new interest is being welcomed by the medical profession because it reduces the harmful effects of everyday life and provides the body with an "break."

What exactly is water Fasting?

Now that you know a more background to fasting, let's go more in depth regarding Water Fasting. In essence, water fasting is a different kind of fasting which only permits you to drink water. They typically last anywhere from 24 hours up to 72 hours. In this period one does not take in any kind of food items and consumes only water.

It is highly recommended not to fast more than the time of 24 to 72 hours , unless you are able to obtain medical approval and are under supervision.
What makes someone want to go on a fast for that length of time? There are many motives for why someone would choose to go fasting and only drink water. These are the reasons:

* For the purpose of a religious ceremony.
* For reasons of spirituality
* To rid the body of toxic substances
* To reap the health benefits of fasting, click here.

* In preparation for a medical procedure operation

A lot of people opt for a the water fast to reap its health benefits, but it's also because there are many advantages associated with drinking water fasts, such as decreasing the chance of getting diabetes, cancer and heart-related diseases.

The practice of fasting with water has been proven to stimulate a process known as autophagy, whereby the body is able to breakdown and recycle certain parts of cells that could be harmful. The lemon detox were developed following the fasting with water. The lemon detox fast permits the drinker to drink many times throughout the day, a mix of lemon juice, water and a tiny amount in cayenne or maple syrup added to the mix for at least seven days.

When it comes to water fasting although it has many health benefits, it's not free of risks. In fact, it could be risky when the fast is extended.

What happens during the 24-72 hours during an Water Fast?
In a water fast during a water fast, you are only allowed to drink water, and not eat any type of food or beverages like juices. You must consume at least two to three liters water every day, for a period of 24 and 72 hours.

Do not ever, ever extend the point at which you can fast, without medical supervision. Limiting yourself to a water-only diet for longer than 72 hours could be hazardous for your health and can cause more harm than good.

While fasting during water it's easy to feel weak or dizzy particularly if you're not used to this. In this period, moderate intensity work is recommended, so avoid machines that are heavy, intense exercises, or even intense workouts.

What happens to your body If You Fast?
The initial few hours into the fast are quite normal. Most people can go on without feeling weak or dizzy. It is because the body is in the normal process of taking in glucose and breaking down glycogen. In the majority of cases 25 percent of glucose is absorbed directly by the brain while the rest is used to strengthen the blood cells and muscles.

In between five and six hours, the majority of people are in ketosis. This is dependent on the sugar levels in your bodyand the speed at which you go to ketosis. Some people are more quickly, while others are slower to achieve ketosis. Ketosis is the state of metabolism of the body , where the energy levels are aided by ketones present in your blood. The process involves dissolving fat. This is the time when real fasting starts, and it is the ideal condition for those who fast to lose weight. The state is also attained through a ketogenic food plan that is a low-carb, high-fat diet.

When your body is in ketosis, a variety of things are likely to occur such as that cholesterol is released and uric acids into the bloodstream. This is an important process as it cleanses the body.

In this condition, the majority of sufferers experience headaches, dizziness, skin rashes and fatigue. The less known symptoms include joint pains and muscle pains. After this phase, pain will begin to ease and blood pressure starts to fall. This process is known as calcification. process in which the mucoid plaque and the cholesterol levels in the body, are reduced.

When our consumption of food is reduced, it helps our digestive system get an opportunity to relaxation. However, because digestion can take some time and is not completely interrupted when we are fasting intermittently. The digestion process is only complete rests when we are on a extended fast.

After the initial 6 days of fasting you'll feel hungry in a natural way, and even a little overwhelmed. This can trigger emotions like anger or anger, sadness, or even depression.

If you're on a fast for a long time let yourself manage these feelings when they occur and to tell yourself that what you feel is because of the fasting you're experiencing.

You don't want to spill your emotions on others around you. This is why fasting must be accompanied by meditation. This is because it shifts your mind off the craving and instead puts it on things can be done with minimal physical effort.

Methods that involve water fasting
What are the Stages of Water Fasting
Stage 1
The first phase usually begins with the time you have eaten your last meal, and can last approximately 12 to 48 hours. Before beginning this type of fast, it's

recommended to conduct an appropriate plan before time to ensure that you are able to complete the duration of the fasting time.

The first phase is generally the most difficult stage you'll be required to pass through towards the start of your fast. At this point you'll begin to feel hungry because of your regular meal intervals as your body begins to adjust during this fasting period. It is also common to feel depleted of energy or experience bad mood swings in this time.

The feeling of "low energy" happens when your body adjusts to the fasting phase, and it begins to burn less energy. This means lowering blood pressure and heart rate. The process is known as "gluconeogenesis," and it is a process in which the liver begins to convert amino acids in glucose in order to gain the energy needed to perform its essential bodily functions.

Stage 2

Stage two starts within the first 48 hours and continues right through seven days. At this point the changes in your appearance begin to appear and you're entering the process called "ketosis." In this point, your body begins to transform the fat within your body into fuel. This is why you may not feel hungry or moody in this time.

Stage 3

The third stage will occur between days 8 and 15 when you begin experiencing changes in your mood. At this point your body has completely in tune with"fasting "fasting" stage and your digestive system enter an "relaxation" stage. Since you've not consumed any solid foods or liquids throughout the past ten days, your body and digestive system will have less work to perform in dissolving food items into bloodstream. If you've reached this stage you'll notice improvements in your general health and energy levels, as well as an increase in concentration.

Stage 4

The day 16 and beyond is the day you are in the fourth stage of your fasting experience. The process will continue toward the end of your fasting time. If you reach this stage you consult with your physician to ensure your continued participation in this phase is under the supervision of your doctor. The fourth stage of the fasting process is the conclusion of the cleansing and repairing process in your body which began in the earlier stages. Therefore, the longer you are fasting longer, the more time your body can recover itself.

Stage 5

The time to break a fast is an individual decision and completely on you and your objectives. It is crucial that if you decide to end your fast, you be patient in adjusting to eating solid food. Your digestive system and body require time to adjust to normal after a prolonged period of fasting. It is recommended to gradually return to this through eating soups and veggies as a beginning. Drinking juices of fruit will aid in the rapid-breaking phase.

How to prepare Your Body

Planning is an essential element in the success of completing the water quickly. Therefore, it is essential to begin preparing your body and mind the best possible way for the time. The first and most important thing is that it is crucial to consult with your physician prior to beginning the type of fast. If you are not in good health the dangers that may be incurred will outweigh the benefits obtained from fasting. Additionally, people with health issues like low blood pressure or diabetes, as well as those who are overweight and women who are pregnant should not fast. So, a thorough medical exam to ensure you are of any medical issues prior to doing this kind of fasting is essential.

The period of fasting can trigger numerous changes in your mental state , too. As you'll experience periods of hunger in the beginning stages of the fast, it's essential to prepare your mind for the challenge that lies ahead. Therefore, it is essential to relax in the beginning phases by being aware of and reducing your cravings and mood swings that may result from lower energy levels. Additionally, you may be affected by diarrhea fatigue, headaches, and body odor, due to the process of eliminating toxic substances and waste in your body. To combat these symptoms it is possible to have a break from working to be in a an environment of relaxation and ease into the whole fasting process.

It is recommended to begin the process slowly "detoxifying" the body. Start by eliminating food items like eggs, meats and fish, as well as milk and cheese. Avoid drinking coffee, sweet drinks as well as alcohol. If you smoke it is recommended to reduce your smoking habits before coming to a complete stop prior to the time your fasting period begins. Change your eating habits by eating more raw and nutritious foods, such as fruits, vegetables and grains. You can gradually begin eating smaller portions of food each time you get toward your fasting date.

You could also get your body ready by a few weeks prior to your water fast by using intermittent fasting to prepare your body and help you manage the hunger cravings. A basic four-week program would be:

1. Week One: Skip eating breakfast.

Week 2: Avoid both lunch and breakfast.

Week 3: Avoid all three meals , and be aware of the portions you eat for dinner.

The 4th week of the Water Fast begins!

In the weeks or days before the start in your period of fasting, you'll require a boost in your intake of water so that your body is prepared for the fast and ensure it's properly hydrated. Finally, ensure you are getting sufficient rest and sleep before and during your period of fasting to ensure that your body is restored and well-rested prior to and during your fasting period.

How Long Should You Fast

The typical fasting time could last from one to forty days, based on the goals you intend to accomplish. If you plan to do any fasts lasting more than forty days, you'll need your doctor's permission prior to making the decision. Below is a brief guidelines provided by Dr. David Jockers, a physician of natural medicine, on the length and frequency of fasting , based on your general objectives. For those who are lean or thin who want to decrease inflammation and chronic illnesses generally, aim to fast for three to five days . Then, do this every 2 to 3 months.

For those who are within your normal BMI weight, that are also seeking to lessen inflammation and chronic illnesses, you should set a goal for a period of fasting that's between 4 and 7 days. Repeat this process for every one and one-half to two months. If you're overweight and aren't solely looking to decrease inflammation and chronic illnesses but are trying to shed excessive weight, you should try an extended fast of between five and 10 (or longer) days. You should repeat this procedure every month.

It is crucial to remember that even well being on a long-term fasting with water can help fight illnesses and regulate your body weight and body composition.

Tips to Take Care of Yourself When You Are Moving

Being fatigued and feeling weak in the beginning of the fasting phase are typical, and it will be essential to get ample rest throughout this time. Make sure you have your sleep pattern with the minimum of 7 to 8 hours of sleep each day. If you require a brief time to recharge your batteries in the course of the day, make sure you use it. Don't overexert yourself during this time. Therefore, you might be advised against engaging in any aerobic or weightlifting exercise during this time since it could only increase your appetite levels. Consider low impact exercises like yoga and stretching in the time that you're attempting this fast. It can also be beneficial to go through a massage to make your fast more enjoyable and aid in the process of detoxifying the body.

Make sure you are well-hydrated. Make sure you drink between nine and thirteen glasses of water daily during your time of fasting. Make sure you drink only pure water or choose to drink distillation water. It is also suggested that if you feel dizzy, you take one teaspoon of salt , and then drink it along with 250ml of water. This will help to balance your insulin levels within the body. Regularly drinking water can aid in reducing the cravings for food that you experience, particularly in the first few days of your fast. It is crucial to remember that you should try to break down the intake of water evenly over all day. Do not drink all of it in one go.

Dizziness is another common sign that can be experienced by those who have been fasting. It usually happens when you rise too quickly. Try to slowly rise to keep from the sudden rush of blood towards the forehead. Deep breathing can assist in stopping this reaction. It is best to lie or sit down if you start to feel dizzy. Relax until the dizziness passes. If symptoms do not go away and become worse, you should stop your fast and consult a physician about your situation. Walking with your feet on dirt or grass can also be beneficial at this phase. By allowing your body's electromagnetic current to be grounded to the Earth by allowing it to ground itself into the Earth, you are giving the healthy electromagnetic frequency emanating from the Earth to flow through your body and function as a kind of antioxidants.

If you are in a warmer environment, you can choose to wear socks instead of walking solely barefoot. This can help improve your mental clarity and assist in relaxing during the fasting phase. Keep a journal during your fasting period can assist you with your mental state during your success in completing the fast. Noting down every day how your body's changes as well as how you feel and the food you consume can help keep your focus on the process and help you stay on the right track.

Other small actions that you can try during this time are these:

* Use a dry brush after you shower (two up to 4 times per daily) to allow the skin to flush out toxic substances. It is also recommended to bathe within warm waters to help open the pores on the skin.

* Make use of activated charcoal to brush your teeth as well as your tongue, as bad breath is typical when you fast for extended durations.

Make sure that you have proper ventilation in the room you're in since body odor is a major issue while fasting.

How to Make Water Fast Fast
How long should you water Fast?
When you're considering water fasting it is the most frequently asked-for solution. The ideal fast is three days, which is ideal for a weekend-long fast. There are however other lengths of standard that could be considered. Whichever length you pick you should give it some careful consideration to it, and must consult with your physician regarding it prior to attempting this type of fast , or any other type of fast.

If you've never had the chance at fasting before taking a couple of hours per day can allow you to become familiar with the feeling and process. The first time you fast, it will provide you with an idea about how you body is able to cope with eating a strict diet. You must learn more about your body's needs by doing the process on your own since every person is unique.

Transition Periods

It is important to keep in mind that the actual duration of the fast is shorter than the commitment for getting your body into the point of being fasting. It is typically referred to as transitional periods that occur before or after the fast in which you take a shower to get rid of a complete diet, and then gradually ease back into your normal eating habits.

The duration of the transition is based on the duration of the fast. It is recommended to cut less than the total number of days during the fast as your transition time. What you're doing is to increase the number of days between start and end. For instance, if you are on a fast over 10 days you must take on a total of 20 days of total attention. A three-day fast would basically require six days of commitment and attention.

For the majority of people, they consider that 4 days are enough to allow for a transition before and following a long fast.

It is, of course, contingent on your goals after the fastand whether you'll adhere to a healthy eating regimen or will be returning to a food-crash habit?

If you're trying the three-day fasting period You should allocate at least a full day before and after the period to transition. Think about how a warm-up and cool-down workout can benefit your body? The transitioning process also works similarly.

For instance, a 3 day fast will require two days before and after the fast. Remember that the longer you wait to adjust your body prior to your fast, the more comfortable your fast will be.

Start by cutting down on the amount of food you consume or perhaps going on a fast for a few hours every day.

How to choose the length

What is the best duration of time to be fasting for you?

The length you choose for fasting should always be the appropriate duration for you at the time you're contemplating it. It is important to not be rigid and flexible throughout your fast, as there are many things that could occur to your body that will require you to stop your fast and eat immediately, for example, if you develop sick or having a stomachache. You may rethink your diet slightly if you experience discomfort or pain and consume small portions of fresh fruit.

It is also important to be aware of your goals prior to starting your fast to ensure that you are ready for the challenge. Also, you shouldn't try to do this repeatedly. Your body needs time to build up its reserves of nutrition after an eating fast.

The recommended time for fasting for body maintenance and balance includes one working day per week, or three days per month, or 10 days in a year.

The most common lengths used for fasting
* One week of fasting This is usually used as a quarterly cleanse detox.
* 10-day fast is among the most well-known options for fasting and this is the typical period of fasting that is

recommended by the master cleanse detox program. A lot of people choose to use this fast for an annual cleanse and detox process.

In essence, the time frame for your fast is contingent on your goals that you wish to achieve:

1. Three-day water fasts help in eliminating toxic substances and cleanses blood

2. Five-day fast - rejuvenates and strengthens your body's immunity system

3. Ten-day fast prevents the occurrence of health issues and can prevent diseases such as an illness that causes degeneration.

Begin Your Fast Beginning with a Supervised Fast

The documentary that was made in 2016 , titled "The Science of Fasting it examines research and issues about penguins who went on a fast for 3-4 months at the same time. The documentary also discussed the effect of the fast on rodents, as studied by scientists in California. While the film may be boring, it could assist to learn more about the advantages and benefits of fasting.

If you are beginning your water-based fast, it is important to think about doing a controlled fast, particularly if the intention is to ease serious illnesses and ailments.

Fasting during the water cycle can be risky and it is crucial to remember that you can only perform it for a maximum time of 72 hours. The most frequent and significant issue with drinking water fasting is the possibility of sustaining injuries from vomiting.

If you are following a controlled fast it is possible to have tests completed prior to starting fasting to make sure that you don't have any health concerns or physical ailments that could make it difficult to complete the fast.

Fasting with supervision is beneficial particularly for people who are overweight and who want to shed weight quickly. Obesity comes with many problems, and a majority of people have a form of addiction or a severe eating patterns.

Another reason to have your fast monitored is to make sure that you don't have emotional attachments to your food. Be careful not to encourage a habit which could result in the development of an eating disorder. Instead, you should fast in order to help promote a healthier lifestyle as well as more healthy eating habits.

How do you find someone to supervise your water fast

You might not have specific health problems that could affect your fast, however, it's never hurts to have your fast monitored, particularly if it is the first time you've done it.

It is possible to ask a medical professional to help you through the fasting process by going through the duration and discussing with you any questions or concerns and also keeping an eye on you during the time you are doing the fast.

Experts who supervise fasts regularly are aware of the changes that your body undergoes and the way they react to fasting. They will be able to provide strategies that are best suited to your requirements. They are also competent to guide you in case fasting isn't worth doing to your body.

The majority of experts will ask that you attend their retreat centers or clinics However, there are some that provide their services through YouTube or Skype which allows you to be fasting from your home. If you are suffering from a particular medical issue, you will be recommended by experts in fasting or your supervisors to see your doctor on a regular basis to make sure your body's vitals are in good condition.

If you are unable to locate an appropriate fasting manager or retreats, clinics, or retreats in your local area, an alternative is to consult your physician regularly and ask whether they can oversee your health while taking a water-only fast.

Medical doctors aren't really experienced with fasting , and might advise you not to practice it.

Goin' at It Alone

While having a professional by your side can help you with the water fasting process, many have successfully attempted it by themselves. In these situations the rational mind as well as an intuitive understanding of your body can aid you in determining when you're doing too excessive and keep you out of danger. Avoid eating more than you can chew. So in the event that you are attempting this for the first time doing it, don't try a 3-day water-fast immediately. Begin by doing a shorter one-day fast which is more comfortable, or try intermittent fasting. You can break the fast with light foods like juices and fresh fruit.

It may be beneficial to start a cleanse one or two weeks before your water fast particularly if you aren't eating well. This will allow you to eliminate any toxins prior to the actual fast and avoid making your body overloaded.

The experience gained during your fast like the body's reaction to emotional triggers that you could experience throughout your fast can be useful in gaining knowledge about your body, and what is required to fast.

It is possible that a three days of water fasting is not suitable for you and you could be stuck with once every week water fasts. These short bursts are informative for you and can help clarify your relationship with food, making it more enjoyable.

Fasting, in its various forms, is a wonderful personal present to us. If you do not want to adhere to long-term fasts then keeping to short-term fasts will benefit your body to heal over time. If you decide to go on a water fast by yourself, then you have to adhere to the rules of fasting, which include recovering and resting.

It is important to take a step back and be mindful of the demands of your body and the messages it's transmitting to you. Fasting can help heal at all levels-physically, mentally, and emotionally. only you will know what you need to do.

The water fast isn't a fool, so be sure to be open to new ideas and be open to change. You should read all you can be aware of the advantages, adverse effects , and other factors that are involved when you fast on water.

Be aware that you aren't trying to compete with anyone else. It is your body, so you must only run the time you are able to and as long as advised to be safe.

The ability to listen to your own internal signals and guidance is essential when you are fasting and do not allow yourself to be influenced by the notion that others are watching you.

Strategies to Stay Healthy How to Stay Healthy During the Fast

Here are a few quick suggestions to help you maintain a healthy and secure fast:

1. Maintain a short fasting period

If you are your first time going on a fast make the duration as short as you can. Keep in mind that there isn't person you're competing with. Start by doing shorter fasts before stepping into a complete day of fasting.

2. Consume a small amount on Fast Days

If you feel you're about to faint , and drinking water isn't helping, then take tiny portions of food to keep you hydrated during your days of fasting. It'll do more good than harm.

3. Keep Hydrated

Of course, fast water requires water. Drink water regularly and as often that you are able to. If you ever feel you need electrolytes add some lemon juice into your bottle of water.

4. Meditate

Meditation can help the body and mind to concentrate and become one. Meditation can help stay away from eating and particular cravings. An hour of meditation each day will help you to relax and keep your attention on your mind and focused on your goal of fasting.

5. Don't break your fasts with the Food

If it's time to end your fast, try not to take a huge quantity of foods. Start with a small amount, like an apple or a glass of milk, or even fruit juice is helpful. This stops the body from experiencing shock.

6. Avoid Fasting if You Are Feeling Unwell

If you feel that you are unable to sustain yourself and you are constantly feeling dizzy, start coughing, or you feel like there is a fever coming on and you need to you should stop. It is not a good idea to fast in case you're sick.

7. Consume a lot of whole foods on non-fasting days

One way to maintain the next fasting period is to eat whole food as eating balanced and healthy food choices can help reduce cravings for sugar and carbs , and also help you build a better taste.

8. Keep Exercise Mild

You may exercise during your fast, however, should you choose to do so, you need to keep it simple. Yoga or meditation, stretching and even a bit of running around in a brisk pace can be helpful.

Benefits of a water Fast and Weight Loss Benefits

Fasting is a notion that has been in use for many thousands of years however, water-based fasting is fairly new. It might appear to be a nigh impossible notion to imagine that the human body could endure for an extended period just on water, however, if you do it with care, it's feasible. In addition, there are numerous benefits and advantages, which include weight loss, which can be derived from it too.

It's no surprise that fasting has been around for longer than it has because of the numerous advantages associated with this type of practice. By fasting with water it is a way of limiting your intake to water only. It's the only thing your body can consume during the process. It doesn't matter if it's 24 hours or 72 hours, in the time you've committed to the water-only fast your body isn't going to experience anything other than a continuous consumption of water.

Water is the life-force of everything on earth. This includes the human body. 60 percent of our bodies are made up of water. It is this vital important element that to keep our bodies alive. Water circulates throughout the cells within our body, our tissues and organs, assisting us maintain the bodily functions we require as we move about our day. We require water to stay alive. Apart from helping with all the bodily functions, it is also essential to keep our digestive system healthy. If we're taking water regular basis, why would you need to drink water quickly?

How did this approach been so popular in recent years? Because of the benefits that are attributed to this method, along with the advantages to losing weight with it. Although some weight loss can be experienced in almost every fasting technique which is consistently followed Water fasting is more than weight loss. It's about overall health.

The benefits of water Fasting

If you're considering beginning the water fasting technique to improve your health you'll be happy to learn that you're likely to enjoy these benefits:

It may help in Autophagy Promotion. Healthline.com is an online health and health publication, reported that a number of studies have revealed that water fasting can aid in the development of autophagy within your body. Autophagy occurs when the older cells within your body are degraded and recycled. This could aid in protecting you from certain diseases, like cancer, heart disease, or Alzheimer's, for instance. Autophagy can help to prevent damaged cells from growing unhealthily within your body. This reduces the risk factors linked to cancer and decreases the likelihood of cancer cells forming. But, there's no enough research done to determine the effectiveness of water fasting in terms of autophagy-promoting and more research in this area is necessary.

It could help lower your blood pressure. A study that was published by NCBI found that following studies, long-term water fasts that are done under medical supervision can help people suffering from hypertension. The same study also revealed that 68 people experiencing excessive blood pressure and were under medical supervision when they ate a diet of water for 14 days (almost). When they had reached the conclusion of their fasting time it was evident the fact that 82% the people noticed a dramatic change of their blood pressure that had decreased to levels that were significantly healthier. Another study was conducted with an entire group of 174 people suffering from high blood pressure. The study experienced the water fasting procedure over a period of between 10 and 11 consecutive days. When the study was over, period 90% of those who were surveyed experienced a decrease in blood pressure to 140/90mmHg. There haven't been enough studies to establish if the same result could be achieved using short-term water fasts or high blood pressure (where fasts vary between 24 and seventy-eight hours).

It may improve the susceptibility to insulin and leptin. The metabolism of the human body is influenced by two crucial hormones, namely the insulin and leptin. This time, NCBI revealed research water fasting may result in the body becoming more sensitive to insulin and leptin. This implies that these hormones will become much more efficient. The increased insulin sensitivity indicates that your body will be more effective in reducing blood sugar levels, and improved leptin sensitivity aids your body to cope with and process hunger signals. Effectively managing your hunger signals and effectively will lower the likelihood of being overweight.

It can help to reduce inflammation in your body. According to research carried out at Yale School of Medicine. Yale School of Medicine, found that fasting can reduce inflammation and proinflammatory cytokines inside your body. It can also help lessen the damage that oxidative causes in the body. The study conducted by Yale School discovered that the hydroxybutyrate (BHB) substance blocks NLRP3 which is component of a family of proteins referred to as an inflammasome. It is responsible of the inflammasome response the body produces in various diseases. These include Alzheimer's disease, autoimmune disease heart disease, and Type two diabetes. What they discovered is that BHB was produced best through fasting, which is probably the most efficient method. Other options include exercise with high intensity, ketogenic diet and reduction in calories.

It could help boost the Immune System of your body. The University of California Professor of Gerontology and Biological Sciences, Dr. Valter Longo who conducted a study in 2014 found that a 3-day water-based fasts can aid in the regeneration of your body's immune system. Fasting allowed the body to activate its regenerative switch and then stimulated stem cells to enter their regenerative state and generate new white blood cells. According the Dr. Longo, tells the body that it's OK to continue with the process of proliferation and rebuild the system. A study conducted by University of California Berkeley University of California Berkeley also supported this by research which revealed that a 3-day water fast is what your body needed to to reset its immune system, allowing to perform at the highest level.

It helps your body reset itself. It's not a surprise that we are subjected to unhealthy foods and lifestyle choices in the present. Foods that are processed, fast food food as well as fatty and processed foods all of it. we've all eaten at one point or another. Many people might even consume more than they need to because of their busy, hectic lives. That is the reason it's important for us to aid our bodies to reset often and the water fast is among the most effective ways to achieve this. It is the one thing that's 100% safe for our bodies, with no negative side effects, as a number of other liquids and foods could cause.

Weight Loss Benefits from Fasting with water Fasting

Here's the most important question for those who are determined to lose weight will want to answer: will drinking water fasting help in weight loss?

Yes however, there's a distinction between burning fat and losing weight. The water fast is not likely to aid you in this, so the bulk of the weight loss you experience will be due to the body's loss of the water, muscle mass and weight through the fast, and carbohydrates. It's not so much about burning fat. It takes a few days for our bodies to begin using its stored fats as fuel If you're looking for an effective fasting for fat burning technique, a different method might work better for you.

But this doesn't mean that there isn't any weight loss likely to occur. There's a certain amount of weight loss advantages you can expect to experience when you drink water fast, particularly in the event that you stick to it for a long time. Different bodies have different processes, which means that some people have a higher level of weight loss in comparison to others. When you follow the water-fast approach, the first stages will involve the loss of weight loss due to water, while fat burning will kick in after your body is deprived of food for a long time.

The chiropractor and acupuncturist in Toronto, Ben Kim, mentions that at the very least, one pounds a day of weight loss could be anticipated when you go through this water-fast (again there is no guarantee that all people's bodies work in the similar way). A few people could lose up to 3 pounds per day, particularly if they've been eating a diet that includes a lot of processed foods in which plenty of water is retained.

If we want to or not, there's no single, guaranteed for weight loss. While water fasting is beneficial to your body, as a whole, is not enough to help in lasting weight loss. According to the Academy of Nutrition and Dietetics suggests the best method to long-term weight loss through the combination of healthy eating and exercise.

A Brief Note of Advice

Similar to any other fasting technique or exercise regimen, or any change of routine, it's advised to consult with your doctor or a health professional prior to beginning a new procedure. A physician who is familiar with your medical history and background will be the best choice in this case since they'll be able to provide you with information about what to be aware of and the best way you can take care of yourself during your fasting time. Discuss with your healthcare professional about your objectives as well as the reasons you're deciding to follow this method of fasting and what you can anticipate. Any time you feel unwell You should take a break and speak with your doctor immediately.

Chapter 9: Pros And Cons Intermittent Fasting With Water Fasting

Whatever you choose to do, you'll discover certain advantages and disadvantages. Knowing these advantages and disadvantages could influence your decision to take on a certain thing or not.

The previous chapter has already shown the benefits of intermittent water fasting. can aid in improving the health of your body and keep it. it may also assist you to shed weight should you wish to.

But, they aren't the only benefits of intermittent fasting in the water:

* Glowing Skin

Food choices could have an impact on how your skin appears. This is due to fats in your food and also the food items that trigger inflammation.

Fasting intermittently will enable you to recognize the foods which are the best for your health and get rid of those that can cause inflammation or other problems. Your well-being will be healthier, which will reflect on your face. Your skin will appear radiant.

In addition, intermittent fasting encourages your body to stay balanced, you'll observe that your nails and hair look better and healthier.

* Spiritual Health

Intermittent fasting is proven to improve your mood. This is due to the fact that it decreases anxiety levels, and also because you're less focussed on finishing tasks so that you can eat.

Being more positive can allow you to appreciate the best things that happen in your life. You will also get a better understanding of the spiritual side and connection to the surroundings that you reside in.

It is vital to note that this is not in any way a belief in faith; religion doesn't require any connection with what you eat.

* Heart Health

The less fat you have in your body, the less likely to be surrounded by fat tissue that will make it more difficult to work. Heart fat can increase the risk of developing heart problems as you get older.

Because intermittent fasting in water aids in weight loss as well as keeping your body in good shape,, it can reduce the amount of fat in your body which will improve the health of your heart.

* Recovery

It is not advised to begin intense exercise while you're fasting. If you're already engaged in an intense workout routine, it might be considered acceptable to keep going. If not, you must start gradually building your fitness routine and pay attention to your body's needs as you go it.

A study has shown that athletes who engage in intermittent fasting may actually see quicker recovery after workouts without losing performance during their workout.

* Cleaning

The practice of fasting in any form can aid your body in its efforts to eliminate any toxins. This is because your body gets the ability to balance hormones, which allows all of your systems to perform at a high level.

With the absence of ne toxins , the proteins as well as other harmful toxins that accumulate within your cells are eliminated. This will lower the chance of getting cancer, Alzheimer's disease and other illnesses that are associated with the aging process.

* Brain Function

It is believed that intermittent fasting can boost the creation of BDNF. This is a nutritional component that is vital to protect your brain against a range of problems.

While it's great to know that intermittent fasting could boost the health of your brain, further research is needed to prove this issue.

* Decline In Hunger

It's as surprising as it may sound it can aid in reducing the hunger cravings. This isn't because you are able to avoid these pangs, or to distinguish between which are really hunger.

The majority of what you eat is just routine. The way you are taught to eat is breakfast lunch, dinner , and tea. Three meals per day.

But, you don't necessarily have to. Fasting intermittently can help you understand your appetite while making sure that your body is getting the nutrition it requires. In a relatively short time of time, your body's body adapts to your food choices without feeling hungry in the time of fasting.

* Extended Lifespan

As mentioned previously, when you're not eating for a prolonged duration, your body will discover a way to live. This is also the case by intermittent fasting. This means that you will increase your longevity!

Advantages

Of course, there is no thing in the universe that's perfect. there will be some negatives to your intermittent fasting plan:

* Special occasions

If you're attending the restaurant, a party, gathering or other occasion, you may be unable to adhere to your fasting schedule.

In actuality, it's simple to begin your slow pace and keep going. In reality every slip marks the first step on an unsteady slope that leaves you wanting to go further but not quite putting the determination to do it.

* Energy Levels

The body requires sugar to provide quick access energy. If you cut out the energy source, your body's metabolism should shift into burning off fat cells.

In the phase of intermittent energy, as you get used to your new sources of energy, you will likely feel exhausted throughout the day. If you're not physically active, you'll probably be struggling to get enough energy to last throughout the working day.

* Eating Over

If you are fasting for 16 hours, you will only have an eight hours to consume food. The thought of this is to motivate you to consume less food and the fat-burning action will significantly increase the effectiveness of your weight loss.

But, in reality, you'll feel at ease to eat whatever you want and this could cause overindulgence.

If you are planning meals and menus that you can precook, this shouldn't be a problem however for a lot of people it will be.

* Dizziness

A lack of blood sugar can cause people to be dizzy. In some cases, you could be able to pass out or fall down when your blood sugar level is low.

The lack of blood sugar could make your brain less able functioning properly, and you could experience difficulties focusing.

This can be addressed by drinking lots of water however it is still a problem which you need to keep in mind.

* Food Cues

The body makes two different hormones to help you get rid of hunger. Leptin is one of them and informs you that you are over-stuffed, effectively stopping your appetite. Ghrelin is the second hormone that signals you that you're hungry.

However, intermittent fasting could cause the hormones to be confused. This means that you will not be able to tell when your body is trying to tell you that it's hungry or in need of food.

* Increased Stress

In fact, not eating will help your body achieve better the balance of hormones. However, long-term periods could actually cause stress because your body is convinced that there's no food in the pipeline and then becomes anxious about it.

The release of stress hormones can cause you to crave food. If you do manage to resist, the added anxiety can make it hard to get a restful sleep.